MULTIDISCIPLINE PATHOLOGY LABORATORY COMPETENCY INTERVIEW PREPARTAION GUIDE

QUESTIONS AND ANSWERS – A TRAINING AND PROFESSIONAL DEVELOPMENT HANDBOOK FOR BIOMEDICAL, HEALTHCARE, MEDICAL LABORATORY SCIENTIST OR TECHNOLOGIST JOB INTERVIEW PREPARATION, ASCPI EXAMINATION, AND OTHER PATHOLOGY LABORATORY INTERVIEW PREPARATION.

DR. EMMANUEL OGBODO
(B.MLS, MSc, PhD, HCPC, FIBMS, FHEA)

Introduction

Preparing for a pathology laboratory interview such as Biomedical Scientist (BMS), Medical Laboratory Assistant interview can sometimes feel overwhelming, especially when you are not sure what questions to expect or how to answer them confidently. This guide has been carefully written to support you - whether you are newly qualified, applying from overseas, or looking for promotion within your current role.

The goal of this book is simple: to help you understand interview questions, structure your answers effectively, and connect your knowledge to practical laboratory experience. Each question is presented with context, key points to consider, and clear, well-structured answers supported by real-life examples from various pathology departments.

Remember, interviewers are not only testing what you know but also how you apply that knowledge in real situations. Try to picture yourself in the laboratory as you answer. This will help you structure your thoughts naturally and speak with confidence.

This book is more than just interview preparation. It aims to help you develop into a reflective, competent, and confident Biomedical Scientist who can communicate ideas clearly and demonstrate genuine passion for laboratory practice.

General Disclaimer

While this guide covers a wide range of potential interview questions, please note that interviewers may ask questions in different ways, or use alternative wording not included in this book.

This book is designed to increase your confidence and improve your chances of success, but it does not guarantee a particular interview outcome.

Aim

The aim of this manual is to equip you with the confidence and understanding to answer interview questions effectively, regardless of the result. The focus is on developing your ability to explain concepts clearly, connect theory to practice, and show professional competence throughout your responses.

Recommendation

Pathology is an evidence-based and highly practical profession. When answering interview questions, it is important to demonstrate both your theoretical knowledge and your understanding of how things work in practice.

The people interviewing you are often experienced laboratory professionals, so always try to connect your answers to real laboratory processes. Use examples from your experience or training that show you understand how to apply your knowledge.

A good way to structure your answers is to think in three stages: pre-analytical, analytical, and post-analytical.

For example, if you are asked:

"What is Quality Control (QC)?"

You can structure your answer as follows:

- Define QC.
- Mention the two types of QC - Internal and External (e.g. NEQAS in the UK).
- Link QC to the Quality Management System (QMS).
- Give practical examples of how QC is performed in the laboratory.

If you do not yet have hands-on experience in the country where you are being interviewed, that is perfectly fine. You can show understanding by referring to your education, training, or transferable skills. For example:

"Although I don't yet have direct experience working as a Biomedical Scientist in the UK, my education and training have equipped me with a solid understanding of key laboratory processes, including quality control, result validation, and sample integrity checks."

Finally, remember that interview panels often award marks for clear, structured answers. A strong response gives points, explains each point briefly (**See table below - Target point 9**), and may include a short scenario to show practical understanding.

In the UK, examples often refer to regulatory bodies such as HCPC, IBMS, MHRA, UKAS, NEQAS, and HTA. If you are outside the UK, simply replace these with your local regulatory authorities or professional titles.

Table: Interview Score.

Score	**1**	**2**	**3**	**4**	**5 (Average)**	**6**	**7**	**8**	**9 (Expectation)**	**10**

Final Note

Interviews are not just about testing your knowledge - they are opportunities to show your commitment, curiosity, and professionalism. Every question is a chance to demonstrate how you think, how you solve problems, and how much you care about the quality of laboratory service and patient care.

Take confidence in what you already know and use this book as a guide to strengthen your answers. Remember, you are not just preparing for an interview; you are preparing for a rewarding career in pathology, where your work will directly impact patient lives every single day.

Question 1:

Tell me about ISO15189 and why follow it in the lab.

Points to consider:

When answering this question, make sure to address the following:

- What is ISO?
- Why 15189?
- Where ISO15189 can be applied - note that other ISO codes exist (e.g., ISO17025, for research laboratories), so differentiate your answer accordingly.
- Applicability to medical (clinical pathology) laboratories.
- Implications of ISO15189 for overall laboratory quality assurance.
- Connection between ISO15189 and your country's accreditation body (for example):
  - UK → United Kingdom Accreditation Service (UKAS)
  - Australia → National Association of Testing Authorities (NATA)
  - Canada → Standards Council of Canada (SCC)
  - (Adjust for the country where you are being interviewed)

Using these points ensures you stay structured and avoid muddling your answer.

Answer:

Thank you for this question. ISO15189 is vital in pathology laboratories because it sets standard policies and guidelines that laboratories must follow to meet international standards.

ISO stands for the **International Organization for Standardization**, and the code **15189** specifically applies to medical laboratories. The purpose of ISO 15189 is to ensure laboratory standards are consistent and reliable worldwide, regardless of where tests are performed. Each country enforces ISO standards through its national accreditation body, promoting uniformity and high-quality performance across laboratories.

ISO15189 functions as a quality management system, ensuring accuracy, reliability, and consistency of results. Its benefits include:

- Improving patient safety through reliable results.
- Enhancing the confidence of biomedical scientists, medical laboratory staff, and healthcare professionals.
- Increasing trust in laboratory processes from patients and regulatory bodies.
- Providing opportunities to improve laboratory processes and risk management.
- Facilitating international recognition and accreditation.
- Ensuring laboratories meet legal and regulatory requirements.

Example: ISO15189 requires that quality control of processes and systems is carried out before running any patient samples. It explicitly states that it is unsuitable to run patient samples if the quality control fails. This ensures results are accurate and consistent with the patient's condition. A passed quality control gives confidence that results are reliable.

You can provide additional examples relevant to your specialty, such as:

- Performing regular equipment maintenance and calibration.
- Ensuring staff are trained and competent to carry out tasks.
- Investigating pre-analytical and analytical factors that may affect results.

Summary:

ISO 15189 is the international standard that ensures medical laboratories deliver accurate, reliable, and consistent results. Regulatory bodies such as **[insert relevant body: UKAS, NATA, or SCC]** enforce these standards to ensure laboratories remain compliant. For example, ISO 15189 requires that all laboratory tasks are performed by trained, competent, and confident personnel, ensuring both patient safety and the quality of laboratory results.

Notes for candidates:

- Link examples to your specialty where possible.
- Emphasize understanding of ISO15189 rather than memorising lengthy definitions.
- The summary version – is for someone that want a concise answer in the interview.

Note: Apply throughout - I would suggest saying "Thank you" at the end of your answer.

Question 2:

Can you tell us about your self

Points to consider:

Before a job advert is published in the public domain (e.g., NHS Jobs), the employer has already created a person specification. That is what you should focus on when answering this question.

When reviewing the job specification, you are likely to see the following points, which I would like you to consider:

- Passion leading to your degree (e.g., BSc in Biomedical Science, Medical Laboratory Science, or Medical Laboratory Technology).
- Qualifications (BSc, MSc, or others).
- Working experience and areas of competence.
- Skills developed while studying or working.
- Alignment with the Trust's values, vision, and mission (where applicable).

These points will help you stay focused when answering. A structured response gives the panel confidence that you fully understand what you are saying.

At this point, pause and check the person specification for the job you are preparing for. If possible, also check the Trust or company's values, vision, and mission, as that will strengthen your answer.

Answer:

Thank you for the question and thank you for the opportunity to interview for this post.

Growing up, I saw the impact that effective laboratory diagnosis can have on patient management. I also witnessed how misdiagnosis, sometimes caused by errors in the lab, led to the loss of loved ones. These experiences ignited my passion to become part of the team that contributes to accurate diagnosis and effective patient care.

This passion led me to pursue a degree in Biomedical Science (please specify your exact degree title, e.g. *Medical Laboratory Science* or *Medical Laboratory Technology*). I completed my degree in [insert degree], and I also hold [insert MSc or other relevant qualifications].

After my degree, I successfully completed my registration portfolio (in some countries this may be referred to as internship; adjust as appropriate). This enabled me to register as a Biomedical Scientist with the HCPC (or the equivalent regulatory body in your country).

Since gaining registration, I have accumulated over [insert number of years] of experience working as a Biomedical Scientist in pathology laboratories. My work has covered a range of specialties, including [specify specialty: Immunology, Biochemistry, Histopathology, Microbiology, Haematology, Blood Transfusion, etc.].

Working in the laboratory has helped me build extensive competence across the following stages:

Pre-analytical:

- Identifying clotted, diluted, old, haemolysed, icteric, or lipaemic samples.
- Detecting sample contamination or incorrect collection methods.
- Understanding how improper sample storage or preparation can affect results.

Analytical:

- Recognising random and systematic errors.
- Detecting issues caused by faulty analysers or operator oversight.

Post-analytical:

- Validating results by checking patient records, diagnoses, or medication history.
- Ensuring results are consistent with clinical presentation before authorisation.

Technical:

- Competent in the use and application of analysers.
- Skilled in troubleshooting, maintenance, calibration, and method validation.
- Performing quality control and interpreting QC results (e.g., Levey-Jennings charts, Westgard rules where relevant).

For **senior-level candidates**, I recommend also highlighting supervisory experience, involvement with UKAS accreditation/ISO15189, appraisals, staff training and competency sign-off, and contributions to service improvement at departmental meetings.

In addition to my technical background, I have developed strong skills, including:

- Multitasking.
- Excellent communication (e.g., English or other languages).
- Teamwork and flexibility.
- Prioritising workload effectively.
- Problem solving and attention to detail.
- Strong IT/computer skills.
- Maintaining confidentiality.
- Adhering to Trust policies and procedures.

Finally, I researched the Trust values before applying. I found that values such as [insert Trust values, e.g., compassion, excellence, care] completely align with my professional values of [insert your values, e.g., integrity, accountability, teamwork].

This alignment is very important to me, as it reassures me that I can thrive in this environment while contributing positively to patient care and laboratory quality.

Summary:

I am a Biomedical Scientist with a degree in [insert degree] and registration with [insert regulatory body, e.g., HCPC]. I have over [insert years] of experience working in [specialty], where I have developed competencies in result validation, analyser use and troubleshooting, and quality control.

I also bring strong skills in teamwork, multitasking, IT proficiency, and problem-solving, all of which I believe are highly valuable to this role. Most importantly, the Trust's values of [insert Trust values] align closely with my own professional principles, motivating me to contribute meaningfully as a member of your team.

Note for candidates without experience:

If you do not yet have direct experience, do not be discouraged. Instead, focus on transferable skills you have gained through your education or other roles, and show a clear understanding of what happens in the laboratory. For example:

"Although I have not yet worked as a Biomedical Scientist, my education and training have equipped me with a strong understanding of laboratory processes, including result validation and quality control. I also developed skills such as problem solving, teamwork, and IT proficiency, which I am confident will help me adapt quickly to this role."

Demonstrating your knowledge and willingness to learn will reassure the panel that you are trainable and motivated.

Question 3:

Take us through your education and experience

Points to consider:

First, I want you to know that this question is almost the same as question number 2. The only difference is that the focus here is on education and experience.

- Education qualification (s) alignment to the person of specification
- Experience gained that support the person of specification.

You can see that you could use your answer for question 2 here and expand further. That would be my recommendation. However, let's focus on what is specifically asked.

Answer:

Thank you for this question. While growing up, I noticed that the pathology laboratory contributes greatly to overall patient wellbeing. In many cases, diagnosis remains vague until accurate laboratory results are obtained that are consistent with the patient's condition. I observed that until then, patients may be misdiagnosed or managed inappropriately. This experience ignited a passion in me to be part of the team that contributes to effective and accurate diagnosis. This led me to study sciences and eventually obtain a degree in Biomedical Science (remember to specify your own degree title but always emphasise that it is consistent with the country where you are being interviewed).

I successfully completed my registration portfolio (commonly referred to as an "internship" in some countries outside the UK), which enabled me to register with the HCPC as a Biomedical Scientist. Following registration, I continued to work in pathology laboratories for over [X years], specialising in [insert specialty if applicable], where I further developed my technical expertise and professional competence.

While working as a Biomedical Scientist in [specialty, e.g. Haematology and Blood Transfusion, Biochemistry, etc.], I have developed extensive experience in result validation (also referred to as result release or authorisation). I have a good understanding of the factors that may influence laboratory results, ranging from pre-analytical to post-analytical. For example:

- Sample issues such as contamination, clotting, dilution, or ageing.
- Wrong sample tube type used
- Wrong patient sample in tube
- Patient-related factors such as medication or underlying condition.

In addition to identifying these factors, I am also competent in investigating whether they have influenced the patient's results. For example, I have contacted the ward in cases of suspected contamination or dilution to clarify how the sample was collected. A sample taken from a drip arm is likely to be diluted, while one taken from a PICC line may be contaminated. Both of which could lead to false results.

Please note: The examples provided here are not exhaustive, so I recommend reflecting on and preparing examples that are most suitable to the specific interview you are attending. Some are already mentioned in question number 2.

I look forward to bringing this passion, my scientific background, and my experience to your team, while continuing to grow by learning from more experienced members of staff.

Summary:

I chose to pursue Biomedical Science because I recognised early on the crucial role accurate laboratory diagnosis plays in effective patient care. I obtained my degree in [state your degree] and successfully completed my registration portfolio (or internship, depending on the country), which enabled me to register as a Biomedical Scientist. Since then, I have gained [X years] of experience working in [state specialty, e.g. Haematology and Blood Transfusion, Biochemistry, etc.].

Through this, I have developed strong skills in result validation, recognising pre-analytical, analytical, and post-analytical factors that can influence results, and troubleshooting laboratory equipment. My background has given me a solid foundation in ensuring accuracy, reliability, and quality in laboratory services.

I believe this combination of education, registration, and hands-on experience makes me well prepared to contribute effectively to your laboratory team.

Question 4:

Why did you apply for this post?

This question aligns with the previous ones. Just because a question is framed differently does not always mean a completely different answer is required. However, here you should put the core question at the centre of your answer.

If you look carefully, they are indirectly asking whether you have the required qualifications, experience, skills, and values for the role. Therefore, the focus should be on the person specification.

Points to consider:

- Education qualifications, including professional membership
- Experience and competencies
- Skills
- Alignment with the Trust values, vision, and mission.
- Location and Specialty

Answer:

I was particularly enthusiastic and excited when I saw this position advertised. One of the main reasons I applied is because I have always wanted to work in this great institution, especially as it is located at the heart of [specify the city]. The hospital is also well known for its significant role in ensuring the wellbeing of women and children (please adjust this based on the actual specialty of the hospital).

This resonates strongly with me, as I have a passion for contributing to the health and wellbeing of women and children, and I feel particularly drawn to children. I also applied because the role matches my professional competency, and I am excited about the combination of the hospital's specialty and location.

I hold a degree in Biomedical Science (with additional qualifications such as an MSc, where applicable) and am a HCPC-registered Biomedical Scientist, meeting the requirements of this position. In addition, I bring several years of experience working in [specify area, e.g. Microbiology, Biochemistry, Haematology, Blood Transfusion, Histopathology, etc.], where I have developed both strong technical expertise and a commitment to maintaining high laboratory standards.

Over this time, I have developed a wide range of competencies. For example, I am confident in results validation, and proficient in the use and application of analysers, including troubleshooting when required. I can also perform analyser maintenance, calibration, validation, and quality control, including interpretation using Levey-Jennings charts and Westgard rules (note: Levey-Jennings and Westgard rules may not be relevant in some departments such as Blood Transfusion).

Beyond technical expertise, I have also developed essential skills such as IT and computer proficiency, effective communication, multitasking, teamwork, workload prioritisation, and confidentiality. For example, as a team player, when I identify non-conformances in the lab, I act quickly to rectify them so that the laboratory continues to maintain conformance with UKAS accreditation and ISO15189 standards (or the relevant regulatory body in the country of interview). I also report such issues to senior staff so that the root cause can be investigated and future occurrences prevented.

Finally, one of my central motivations for applying for this role was the hospital's values, such as [insert actual Trust values, e.g., Compassion, Improving Lives, Everyone Counts]. These are completely aligned with my own professional values, such as [state your own values here].

I look forward to demonstrating the qualities I have highlighted if I am given the opportunity to join your team.

Summary:

I applied for this post because it combines my passion, education, and professional competencies with the Trust's vision, mission, and values. I hold a degree in Biomedical Science and am a HCPC-registered Biomedical Scientist with experience in [state specialty], where I developed skills in results validation, analyser use and troubleshooting, and quality assurance. I have also gained strong transferable skills such as teamwork, IT, and problem solving.

Most importantly, I am motivated by the Trust's values of [insert Trust values], which align closely with my own professional values. This makes me confident that I can make a meaningful contribution while continuing to develop my career here.

Question 5:

Why did you choose to work here?

This question is similar to questions 2 and 3 but requires a clearer and more structured approach to ensure you address the key points expected. As mentioned in question 2, it's important to review the Trust's values and align them with your own professional values. This question is precisely why that matters. Every Trust has a vision, mission, and set of core values, and anyone seeking to work with them must demonstrate full alignment and commitment to these principles.

Points to consider:

- Trust values, vision, and mission.
- Trust area of specialty (e.g., Trauma centre, Women and Children, etc.).
- Environment (location, how busy the lab is, how computerised and well-equipped it is).
- Responsibility (how many samples they process daily/weekly/yearly; how busy the lab is; size of the community served).
- Ethics – Equality, Diversity, and Inclusiveness.

The above points demonstrate you have done your research, and you are convinced that the Trust is the ideal place for you to work.

To give us a better picture, let's assume the following (remember this may differ, so research the Trust where you are being interviewed):

- Values – Compassion, improving lives, everyone counts
- Vision - To provide high quality healthcare for all
- Mission – To improve and protect the health of the population
- Specialty – Trauma Centre
- Hospital Location – London
- Environment – Well computerised and busy lab
- Responsibility – Serving 1.5 million people.
- Numbers samples processed per day – 5000

Please remember to adjust your response where the above differs from where you are shortlisted for interview. For example, it may not be as busy as London. The above is just an example.

Answer:

Thank you for this question. I believe it is an important one, as performance at work is often linked to how well an individual aligns with the Trust's values and ethics.

One of my main motivations for applying for this role is the Trust's values: Compassion, Improving Lives, and Everyone Counts. Additionally, the Trust's vision of providing high-quality healthcare for all, along with its mission to improve and protect the health of the population, strongly resonate with me. These principles align closely with my own professional values and beliefs about delivering quality care in healthcare.

In both my previous and current roles (you can specify the role), I have demonstrated these values by contributing to patient care in every way possible. For example, on many occasions I have been asked to cover shifts during staff shortages. I accepted because I understood the impact short staffing could have on patients and colleagues. In the laboratory, I have also gone beyond routine processes to ensure accurate diagnosis. For instance, investigating cases where pre-analytical factors such as sample contamination or dilution may have affected results. Sometimes this meant contacting the ward, and in urgent cases, personally tracking the repeated sample until results were validated.

- This demonstrates my strong alignment with the Trust's values, vision, and mission.

Another motivation for applying is the Trust's status as a major trauma centre, which makes it one of the busiest hospitals in the region. The laboratory serves approximately 1.5 million people and processes around 5,000 samples daily. I believe this environment will provide me with significant opportunities to learn and grow, while also allowing me to contribute to the laboratory's quality and efficiency.

Furthermore, the Trust's commitment to equality, diversity, and inclusiveness appeals to me, as I strongly believe in a workplace where everyone has an equal opportunity to thrive

Lastly, the location in London is ideal for me. London offers not only a vibrant, diverse environment but also excellent transport links and many opportunities for professional progression. I am excited about the possibility of joining a team in such a dynamic city and contributing to improving the lives of the community.

Summary:

I chose to apply to this Trust because its values, vision, and mission, Compassion, Improving Lives, and Everyone Counts, closely align with my own professional principles. Furthermore, the Trust's reputation as a major trauma centre serving 1.5 million people and processing 5,000 samples daily demonstrates that it is a dynamic, busy, and well-equipped environment where I can both contribute and continue to develop professionally. I am also motivated by the Trust's commitment to equality and inclusiveness, as well as the opportunity to work in London, which offers both professional and personal growth.

Question 6:

What makes you the best candidate for this post?

This question is similar to many of the previous questions. To answer it effectively, you should focus on the person specification and explain why your qualifications, experience, and skills make you a strong fit for the role.

Points to consider:

- Academic qualifications
- Professional membership
- Experience
- Skills
- Alignment with the Trust values.

Answer:

In addition to my passion for working as a biomedical scientist, which allows me to contribute to the community's well-being, I hold a degree in Biomedical Science and am HCPC registered, which enables me to practice as a biomedical scientist.

Over the years, I have gained extensive experience relevant to this role. For example:

- I am highly experienced in processing and analysing biological samples, while being aware of factors that can influence results.
- I am competent in investigating factors such as haemolysis, old samples, or EDTA contamination that could lead to false results (e.g., falsely raised potassium). I also take appropriate actions to ensure such results are not released to patients – **This may be more appropriate for biochemistry interview, that is why I recommend expanding examples relevant to department you are being interviewed**.
- I have contributed to training younger or newly qualified colleagues, helping them understand laboratory processes and standards.
- I have been involved in UKAS laboratory accreditation and external quality assurance schemes such as NEQAS.

In addition to my passion to work as a biomedical scientist, which I believe allows me the opportunity to contribute to the community wellbeing. I have a degree in biomedical science, and I am HCPC registered, which allows me to work as a biomedical scientist.

Over the years of working as a biomedical scientist, I have developed several experiences, which are relevant to this role. For example, just to mention a few: I have excellent experience in processing and analysing biological samples. In doing this I am aware of possible factors that may influence this, and I am competent in investigating these factors. For example, in a case of haemolysis, old samples, or EDTA contamination leading to a false raised potassium result. Also, I know the important of taking appropriate actions to ensure that such result is not released to the patients. My experience has allowed me to contribute to the training of younger or newly qualified colleagues. I have also been involved in the UKAS laboratory accreditation and external quality assurance scheme such as NEQAS.

In addition to my experience, I have developed several key skills:

- Excellent communication in English
- Multitasking

- Teamwork
- Attention to detail
- Hardworking
- IT competency, including use of MS Office and laboratory information management systems such as MediTech, LabCentre, Telepath, Bank Manager, Cerna (adjust to your personal skills)

These skills enable me to maintain laboratory quality and minimise errors. **For example:**

While on shift, one analyser stopped working, causing a backlog of samples. I communicated with the ward to request that only urgent samples be sent until the issue was resolved, while simultaneously troubleshooting the analyser, answering calls from clinicians, and phoning results, all without error. This experience demonstrates my effective communication, prioritisation, and multitasking skills.

All of the points I have mentioned align directly with the person specification for this role, which is why I believe I am the right candidate. I am confident that I can contribute to the success of the laboratory while continuing to develop my professional skills.

Furthermore, the Trust values (please specify) completely align with my professional values (please specify), which strengthens my motivation to join this team. I am committed to ensuring that service users receive high-quality services in line with UKAS ISO15189 standards (adjust according to your country).

Summary:

I believe I am the best candidate for this post because I meet all the key requirements outlined in the person specification. I hold a degree in Biomedical Science and am HCPC registered, enabling me to practice as a biomedical scientist.

I have gained extensive experience in processing and analysing biological samples, investigating factors that may influence results, and contributing to training colleagues. I have also been involved in UKAS accreditation and external quality assurance schemes.

In addition, I have developed key skills in communication, multitasking, teamwork, attention to detail, and IT competency, all of which enable me to maintain high laboratory standards and minimise errors.

Finally, the Trust values, vision, and mission completely align with my professional values, and I am motivated to contribute to the team while ensuring high-quality patient services in line with ISO15189 standards.

Question 2 – 6 are ideal for writing job application supporting information (Example template – see appendix)

Question 7:

What actions would you take following a failed Quality Control procedure on an analyser?

Points to consider:

- What is QC?
- Link QC to ISO15189 recommendation
- Importance of QC
- Types of QC: qualitative vs. quantitative
- Link to Quality Management System (QMS) and Quality Assurance (QA)
- Systematic approach to actions

Answer:

Thank you for this question. Quality control (QC) is central in pathology laboratories because it ensures accuracy, reliability, and precision of results, which in turn supports patient safety and effective diagnosis. Under ISO15189, QC must be performed before testing patient samples, and passing QC is key to laboratory accreditation and maintaining the quality management system (QMS).

QC can be:

- **Internal QC** – is a laboratory daily self-check to confirm that processes and equipment are performing within set limits.
- **External QC** – is conducted by external bodies such as NEQAS, comparing the laboratory performance with other laboratories to ensure consistency and accuracy, which then support national quality assurance scheme.

QC also comes in two main types:

- **Qualitative QC** – This checks whether a result is present or absent, positive or negative (common in microbiology or blood transfusion, e.g., antibody screening).
- **Quantitative QC** – This is numerical values that is compared against set limits (common in haematology or biochemistry, e.g., haemoglobin levels or liver function tests).

The type of QC that fails can affect the investigation approach.

Actions I would take:

1. Stop testing patient samples immediately.
2. Review the QC results – identify which parameter(s) failed and whether it was qualitative or quantitative. For quantitative results, I would check Levey-Jennings charts for trends or shifts; for qualitative, I would check if the expected reaction strength matched the control.
3. Investigate systematically:
    - **Personnel:** operator error such as poor mixing, insufficient sample volume, incorrect storage, expired reagents/QC materials, or incorrect lot number.
    - **QC material:** expired, contaminated, degraded due to poor storage, or used beyond stability.
    - **Reagents:** expired, contaminated, bubbles in tubing, wrong lot number, or insufficient volume.

- **Analyser:** maintenance overdue, calibration drift, bacterial contamination in channels, or mechanical faults.

4. **Corrective actions:**
   - Replace QC material or reagents if suspected.
   - Perform analyser maintenance or recalibration.
   - Repeat the QC after corrective actions.

5. **Next steps:**

- **If QC passes:** continue testing, document actions in the event log/handover, and cross-check around 10 recent patient samples against another analyser where possible.
- **If QC fails again:** take analyser out of service, escalate to a senior, and contact the engineer. Ensure all actions and outcomes are documented in the event and handover book.

Examples across specialties:

- **Haematology:** If QC fails for haemoglobin while other FBC parameters pass, I will suspect reagent or channel-specific issues. I will check for clots, blockages, or calibration errors affecting the haemoglobin channel.
- **Biochemistry:** If liver function QC fails for ALP but passes for AST/GGT, I would consider whether the ALP reagent is expired or contaminated, or whether that specific channel needs flushing.
- **Blood Transfusion:** If antibody screening QC gives weaker-than-expected reactions, I will confirm that reagents and QC samples are viable and stored correctly and ensure that incubation steps were followed precisely.
- **Microbiology:** If antimicrobial susceptibility QC fails, I'd review media quality, incubation conditions, or disc potency.

This approach ensures compliance with ISO15189, protects patient safety, and maintains laboratory quality standards.

Summary:

If QC fails, I would stop patient testing immediately and investigate systematically. I would first determine whether the failure was in qualitative or quantitative QC, then review possible causes, such as operator error, QC material, reagents, or analyser issues. After implementing corrective actions, such as replacing reagents, recalibration, or maintenance, I would repeat the QC. If it passes, I would document all steps taken and cross-check recent patient results to ensure accuracy.

. If it fails again, I'd remove the analyser from service, escalate, and contact the engineer. This approach ensures compliance with ISO15189, protects patient safety, and maintains laboratory accreditation.

Question 8:

With the night/weekend shift pattern meaning you may spend less time working alongside the general BMS team, how would you ensure that you maintain up-to-date CPD, training, and competence?

Background:

When working mainly night or weekend shifts, you may not always be present during the day when updates, training sessions, or discussions occur. While being on the shift rota demonstrates that you can work independently, the challenge is maintaining your competence over time. If laboratory processes

Points to Consider:

- **Continuing Professional Development (CPD):** webinars, online training, reflective logs, journals, podcasts, and professional reading.
- **Outstanding tasks:** incident reports, reflective forms, or audit tasks that can be done during quiet periods on shift.

- **Competence maintenance:** keeping up with QMS updates (e.g., Q-Pulse), acknowledging SOP changes, and staying engaged in accreditation/quality activities.
- **Planning and prioritisation:** making time to catch up on training outside shifts if needed.
- **Engagement:** keeping in touch with colleagues and seniors for updates.

Answer:

Thank you for the question. I understand that working mostly night or weekend shifts can sometimes mean less face-to-face contact with the wider BMS team and potentially missing updates or training opportunities. However, I would take several steps to ensure I remain up to date with my CPD, training, and competence.

Firstly, I would make sure I keep up with any changes within the laboratory by checking and acknowledging updates through our Quality Management System (e.g., Q-Pulse). This ensures I am aware of any changes to SOPs, methods, or policies.

Secondly, I would actively manage my CPD by engaging in professional development activities such as attending webinars, reading relevant scientific journals, reflecting on cases, and using resources like HCPC CPD tools. During quieter times on shift, I would also use the opportunity to complete reflective logs or outstanding tasks such as incident follow-ups.

Thirdly, I would plan and prioritise my tasks carefully. For example, where the shift allows, I could dedicate time to reviewing recent updates or completing training modules. I would also ensure open communication with senior colleagues and participate in any scheduled training sessions when on day shifts.

Finally, I see CPD as an ongoing responsibility. By keeping track of my development and consistently engaging with both internal updates and external learning resources, I would ensure that working shifts does not negatively affect my competence.

Summary:

Although night and weekend shifts reduce the opportunity for face-to-face training, I would remain proactive in keeping my competence and CPD up to date. I would regularly review QMS updates such as Q-Pulse, complete any outstanding tasks during quieter periods, and plan ahead to ensure I do not miss training opportunities. In addition, I would engage in continuous CPD activities such as webinars, reading, and reflection. This approach ensures I remain competent, aligned with ISO15189 standards, and compliant with HCPC requirements.

Question 9:

Briefly define Accuracy and Precision, Trend and Bias and give an example of each to clarify your answer

Background:

This question tests your understanding of quality control (QC) interpretation as a quality assurance (QA) tool. In pathology laboratories, ensuring accuracy, precision, and correct QC interpretation (trends and bias) is central to producing reliable and reproducible results. Ultimately, these concepts are tied to ISO15189 requirements and are critical for patient safety because any error in measurement can mislead diagnosis or treatment.

Points to consider:

- Accuracy - closeness to the true value
- Precision - reproducibility of measurements
- Trend - movement of QC results over time on a Levey-Jennings chart
- Bias - persistent shift away from target mean (positive or negative)
- Link all definitions to QA and patient safety

Answer:

Accuracy refers to how close a measurement is to the true value. For example, if the true concentration of a sample is 10 mg, a result of 9.8 mg is more accurate than 9.6 mg. Accuracy is usually assessed using traceable reference standards or QC materials with known values.

Precision, on the other hand, refers to the closeness of repeated measurements of the same sample. For example, testing a sample five times might yield results of 6.5 mg, 6.4 mg, and 6.3 mg. Although these values are far from the true value of 10 mg, they are close to each other, indicating that the method is precise but not accurate. Conversely, results such as 9.9 mg, 9.8 mg, and 9.7 mg demonstrate both accuracy and precision.

Trend refers to how QC results shift over time on a Levey–Jenning's chart. Each QC point is plotted, and the pattern of these points is the QC trend (**See "LEVEY-JENNINGS CHART & WESTGARD RULES" my YouTube Channel @2GoodBmsJobs**). A drift upwards or downwards from the mean may indicate systematic error, often caused by reagent deterioration, analyser faults, or sample instability. Monitoring trends is vital for early error detection.

Bias is a systematic deviation from the target mean. It is often seen as a persistent positive or negative shift in QC results, even if the points remain within acceptable limits. For example, a 1-2S (**See "LEVEY-JENNINGS CHART & WESTGARD RULES" my YouTube Channel @2GoodBmsJobs**) or 1-3S violation in Westgard rules may indicate bias. Common causes include instrument calibration issues or changes in reagent batches. If bias is identified, recalibration and investigation of the analyser or reagents would be necessary.

Summary:

Accuracy refers to how close a result is to the true value, while precision is how reproducible repeated measurements are. For example, a test result of 9.8 mg for a sample with a true

value of 10 mg is accurate, while results like 6.3, 6.4, and 6.5 mg are precise but not accurate. QC trending, usually plotted on a Levey-Jenning's chart, shows how results move over time and helps detect systematic errors such as reagent deterioration. Bias is a persistent shift above or below the target mean, often caused by calibration or reagent issues. Understanding and monitoring these parameters are essential for maintaining ISO15189 standards, ensuring reliable results, and safeguarding patient safety.

Question 10:

Briefly explain what you understand by the calibration of an analytical method and what is the function of quality control. You can provide examples of calibration you have done.

Background:

This question tests your understanding of the role of calibration in ensuring accurate laboratory measurements. Calibration determines how an analyser measures a substance using QC set mean limits, ensuring that the analyser produces reliable results. Calibration correction factors (mathematical adjustments that align analyser readings with the true, known standards) are adjustments applied when the analyser's calculation differs from the known standard. For example, if a glucose analyser consistently reads 5% higher than the true value, the correction factor is applied to bring the result back in line with the expected value. Another example is when changing reagent batches alters the slope or intercept of the calibration curve; the correction factor ensures patient results remain accurate. Quality control helps detect when these correction factors shift, which could affect the calculation of unknown samples, such as patient results.

Points to consider:

- What is calibration?
- Link to QC
- Impact of calibration correction factor on laboratory results.

- Provide simple examples

Answer:

Calibration is a laboratory technique used to ensure that an analyser provides accurate measurements. It involves using a known standard concentration to generate a calibration curve, which the analyser then uses to calculate the concentration of unknown samples, such as patient specimens. Essentially, the analyser cannot measure anything outside the calibration curve range. Therefore, for a patient result to be valid, the measurement must fall within the calibrated range whether it is low, normal, or high.

Quality control plays a critical role in ensuring successful calibration. QC provides a set of mean limits that the calibration must fall within. If the QC results are within these limits, the calibration is considered valid. QC also helps identify when calibration correction factors have changed, which could impact the accuracy of patient results.

Example:

In a biochemistry laboratory, I have calibrated a glucose analyser using a series of standard glucose solutions. The analyser generated a calibration curve based on these standards. Once the calibration was complete, I ran QC samples at low, normal, and high glucose concentrations. The results fell within the QC set mean limits, confirming that the calibration was successful. If the QC results had been outside the expected range, it would have indicated a problem with the calibration, such as a change in the correction factor (for example, the analyser reading 5% higher than expected) or an issue with the reagent, requiring investigation before patient samples could be processed.

Summary:

Calibration ensures that analysers provide accurate measurements by generating a curve from known standards. Quality control verifies that the calibration is valid and helps

detect errors or shifts in calibration correction factors, which could affect patient results. For example, running QC samples after calibration confirms that the analyser is performing within expected limits, ensuring reliable and accurate results for patient care.

Question 11:

Give us an example of when you demonstrated good verbal and written communication.

Background:

This question is testing your communication skills. You are expected to provide practical evidence that demonstrates how you communicate effectively. The question also examines whether you understand that good communication supports accurate and effective diagnosis, while poor communication can negatively impact patient care.

Points to consider:

- Verbal and written communication skills
- Role of communication in accurate diagnosis and patient management
- Being a team player and working collaboratively
- Personal experience demonstrating communication to support accurate diagnosis

Answer:

Pathology is a complex and dynamic environment that relies on teamwork and collaboration with other healthcare professionals, such as doctors and nurses. Effective communication is crucial because the laboratory does not operate in isolation, and any misunderstanding or miscommunication can directly affect patient care and outcomes.

Example:

There have been several occasions where I had to phone a ward regarding a patient's sample integrity. For instance, a sample may have been collected from a drip arm, which could dilute the patient's results. In these situations, I ensure I communicate clearly and effectively, confirming details with the ward staff and advising on sample repetition if necessary, so that an accurate result can be reported.

Similarly, I have received calls from wards with queries about patient results. I always respond in a way that ensures the service user benefits and that patient care is not compromised. For example, I have communicated urgent results multiple times such as high potassium, abnormal INR, or low haemoglobin ensuring the information was communicated clearly and accurately so that immediate clinical action could be taken.

In addition to verbal communication, I document these interactions accurately in the LIMS lab note area, handover notes, and incident forms where necessary, ensuring that written communication complements verbal communication to maintain continuity of care.

Summary:

Effective communication is central to ensuring accurate and timely patient management in a pathology laboratory. I consistently demonstrate good verbal and written communication by interacting clearly with clinical teams and colleagues. For example, when a patient sample appears diluted due to collection from a drip arm, I proactively phone the ward to clarify the collection method, ensuring the sample collection is repeated to ensure that the results reported are accurate. I also communicate urgent results, such as high potassium, abnormal INR, or low haemoglobin, in a clear and concise manner so that clinicians can take immediate action. Additionally, I document all communications, including handover notes, incident forms, and laboratory records, to maintain continuity of care and support quality assurance. This approach ensures patient safety, facilitates effective

teamwork, and aligns with laboratory standards for accurate diagnosis.

Question 12:

What role do you think a Band 5 should play in audit?

Background:

This question is testing your understanding of laboratory audits, including the definition, types, and their link to Quality Management Systems (QMS) and Quality Assurance (QA). Although it specifies Band 5, the underlying expectations often apply across different bands, with the difference being the level of responsibility and extent of involvement. For a Band 5, the focus is usually on participation, developing audit skills, and demonstrating competence, which also supports progression to higher bands.

Points to consider:

- What is audit?
- Audit role in QMS and QA
- Types of audits (internal, external, vertical, horizontal, witness, clinical)
- Audit and competency
- Participation of a Band 5

Answer:

An audit is a structured process within the Quality Management System (QMS) that assesses whether prescribed standards and procedures are being followed. In the pathology laboratory, audits ensure that practices comply with ISO 15189 standards, providing assurance of accuracy, reliability, and patient safety. When evidence shows that standards are met, it builds confidence in the laboratory's processes. Conversely, when standards are not met, non-conformances are identified, triggering investigations, corrective actions, and, where appropriate, additional training.

There are two main types of audits:

- Internal audits, conducted by laboratory staff to monitor compliance with SOPs, policies, and ISO standards.
- External audits, conducted by accreditation bodies such as UKAS (UK), NATA (Australia), or CAP (USA) to independently assess compliance.

Audits can also take different forms:

- **Vertical audit** - following a single sample through its entire journey, from collection to reporting.
- **Horizontal audit** - checking one process across multiple samples or cases (e.g., sample reception).
- **Witness or examination audit** - observing staff performing tasks to confirm competence.
- **Clinical audit** - reviewing laboratory services against clinical outcomes or service user needs.

For a Band 5 biomedical scientist, participation in audits usually begins with supportive roles, under supervision, and gradually develops into more independent tasks as competence grows. Examples of roles include:

- **Internal audit participation:** Reviewing a small section of documentation (e.g., ensuring haemoglobin SOPs are being followed correctly).
- **Vertical audit:** Tracing a transfusion sample from request to reporting, checking every step for compliance.
- **Audit preparation:** Assisting senior staff by ensuring QC logs, analyser maintenance records, and staff competency records are up to date.
- **Closing non-conformances:** Correcting minor issues highlighted in audits, such as ensuring reagent lot numbers are recorded correctly.
- **Witness audit:** Being observed while performing tasks (e.g., analyser calibration or maintenance) to demonstrate competence.

Example:

During an internal audit in the haematology section, I was asked to review maintenance logs for one of the analysers. I identified that while most records were complete, one shift had missed documenting the daily maintenance for two consecutive days. I raised this with my senior, ensured the logs were corrected, and added a note in the handover record. This not only resolved the non-conformance but also reinforced my awareness of the importance of thorough documentation in maintaining ISO15189 compliance.

By participating in these tasks, Band 5 staff contribute to the overall audit process while also developing their own skills in attention to detail, quality awareness, and professional growth.

Summary:

A Band 5 biomedical scientist plays a crucial role in audits by supporting internal processes, preparing and checking records, tracing sample journeys, correcting non-conformances, and participating in witness audits. For example, reviewing analyser maintenance logs or sample records ensures compliance with ISO15189 and helps prevent non-conformances. While not leading audits, Band 5s develop valuable skills, build confidence, and contribute to patient safety while preparing for higher responsibilities in the future.

Question 13:

What is your greatest achievement and why?

Background:

This question is assessing how you reflect on your professional journey, the impact of your contribution, and how your achievements have shaped you as a biomedical scientist. While personal achievements are valid, interviewers are generally more interested in examples directly linked to laboratory practice, patient care, or professional development. Linking your achievements to teamwork, problem-solving, and quality patient outcomes will make your answer stand out.

Points to consider:

- Successful events in the lab where you played a central role.
- How you contributed to patient safety or service improvement.
- How the experience improved your professional confidence and work ethic.
- Personal or academic milestones that enhanced your competence.

Answer:

Working in the laboratory provides a balance of challenges and rewarding moments. Challenges remind me of the importance of continuous improvement, while successes offer strong encouragement. These achievements not only strengthen my confidence but also shape my approach to delivering patient-focused care.

I will now provide some examples, which are not exhaustive and can be applied in a manner consistent with the role I am applying for.

Example:

Haematology/Biochemistry (Technical & Problem-Solving):

One of my greatest achievements occurred while on an early night shift when one of the analysers began giving continuous error messages, disrupting the workflow at a time when urgent ward and A&E samples were building up. It was particularly daunting because I had only recently joined the shift rota independently.

Despite the pressure, I isolated the faulty analyser, prioritised urgent ward samples, and continued processing using the available analyser. Simultaneously, I managed incoming phone queries from wards and GPs, ensuring clear and effective communication. Through systematic troubleshooting, I identified the issue as clot aspiration. After flushing and replacing the probe, I successfully restored the analyser, validated QC, and returned to normal workflow. I consider this a major achievement because the fault was resolved without significantly delaying urgent patient results. This experience reinforced my ability to multitask, prioritise under pressure, and maintain turnaround times in critical situations.

Blood Transfusion (Patient Safety):

Another key achievement was completing my Specialist Portfolio in transfusion science. It equipped me with the skills to investigate transfusion reactions and report appropriately to the MHRA. For example, I successfully contributed to an investigation where a suspected febrile non-haemolytic transfusion reaction required correlation of clerical checks, laboratory serology, and patient history. My role helped ensure the correct clinical recommendations were made, supporting both patient safety and regulatory compliance.

Microbiology/Histopathology (Service Contribution):

In microbiology, I was once part of an internal audit reviewing specimen labelling and transport compliance. My contribution led to identifying recurring pre-analytical issues from specific wards. By presenting findings and suggesting refresher training for ward staff, error rates significantly dropped. In histopathology, a similar achievement was assisting in implementing a new tissue tracking system, which improved traceability and turnaround times for biopsy samples.

Professional Development (Long-Term Achievement):

Another proud moment was successfully completing my MSc degree alongside full-time laboratory work. Balancing both commitments was challenging, but it gave me advanced knowledge in molecular diagnostics and research skills. This achievement not only enhanced my scientific competence but also taught me resilience, discipline, and the importance of lifelong learning.

Summary:

My greatest achievements reflect a balance of technical problem-solving, patient safety, and professional growth. From restoring analyser function under pressure and ensuring critical patient results were not delayed, to completing my Specialist Portfolio and MSc, each achievement has strengthened my confidence and competence as a biomedical scientist. These experiences shaped my ability to multitask, prioritise effectively, and continuously improve, all of which are essential for contributing to high-quality patient care and laboratory service delivery.

Question 14:

Do you have any questions for us?

Background:

When this question is asked, many candidates respond with "no questions." This is not ideal, as it may suggest a lack of research or genuine interest in the Trust or hospital. A strong candidate demonstrates curiosity and engagement by asking thoughtful questions about the organisation, the role, and opportunities for professional development.

If you have researched the Trust, you should be able to ask something around their values, vision, and mission. You can also ask about their shift patterns, training, CPD opportunities, or laboratory strategies to maintain quality and staff wellbeing. Asking thoughtful questions not only demonstrates preparation but also helps you evaluate whether the Trust is the right fit for you.

Points to consider:

- Research on the Trust values, vision, and mission.
- Working/Shift pattern.
- Available Training and CPD.

- Laboratory support structures (mentorship, wellbeing, audits).

Answer:

Thank you for the opportunity to be interviewed. I do have some questions I would like to ask:

- **Trust Values/Quality:** I noticed from my research that one of the Trust's values is safety. What strategies are in place within the laboratory to ensure this is achieved, particularly in relation to maintaining ISO15189 quality standards? (Alternatively, questions can be framed around the Trust's vision or mission).

- **Shift Pattern and Training:** I understand from the job advert that the laboratory provides a 24/7 service. Could you please share how training and competency sign-off are structured to ensure staff are well prepared before joining the shift rota? Also, could you explain what the typical shift patterns are like, including night and weekend coverage?

- **Professional Development:** I am very keen on continuous professional development. Could you outline the types of internal and external CPD opportunities available for staff? For example, are there study days, external courses, or support for attending scientific conferences?

- **Career Progression:** I would also like to know if the Trust supports staff in completing specialist portfolios (such as IBMS Specialist Portfolio) or postgraduate training (e.g., MSc), and whether it is possible to undertake these while working full-time.

- **Other Considerations:** Some candidates also ask about mentorship or wellbeing. For instance: Does the department have a mentorship system in place for Band 5s to support their transition into more senior roles? Or What measures are in place to ensure staff wellbeing, especially for those working frequent night shifts?

These are just examples, but they demonstrate curiosity and preparation. You don't need to ask all of them. I would recommend asking just two or three well thought-out questions.

Summary:

Yes, I do have a few questions. I would like to know how the laboratory ensures its work aligns with the Trust's values, particularly in maintaining patient safety and quality. I am also interested in understanding the training and CPD opportunities available, including whether staff can complete their specialist portfolio while working full-time. Finally, I would like to ask about the shift patterns and how the laboratory supports staff to achieve competence and confidence before moving onto the rota.

Question 15:

Give us an example of when you carried out error logging

Background:

This question acknowledges that errors in the pathology laboratory are sometimes unavoidable. The aim is to test whether you have experience recognising such errors, know how to report them, and understand the role of error logging in improving laboratory systems. It is important to differentiate between different types of errors. For example, equipment or method failures (often beyond staff control) versus individual mistakes (such as a misjudgement during result validation). Both require recording, but the focus here is on systematic errors like equipment, reagents, or procedural issues, which are logged to allow troubleshooting, learning, and prevention of recurrence.

Point to consider:

- What is an error?
- What is error logging?
- Effective ways to log errors.
- Your personal experience with error logging.
- Practical examples appropriate to the department.

Answer:

Errors in the laboratory are defined as deviations from the expected process or outcome that may compromise the accuracy and reliability of results or pose a risk to patient safety. Error logging is the systematic recording of such incidents in accordance with the laboratory's Quality Management System (QMS). This process ensures traceability, supports root cause analysis, and provides documented evidence for implementing corrective and preventive actions.

When an error occurs, the first step is to recognise and troubleshoot it. If resolved, I record the event on the error log and include the corrective action taken, so others can follow the same steps if the issue reoccurs. If unresolved, I still document it clearly, escalate it to the senior team, and ensure follow-up. This log is later reviewed during audits, staff meetings, or updates to SOPs.

Please see examples below and apply them in line with the area you are being interviewed for. Remember, the examples in this manual are not exhaustive. You can adapt or expand them with your own experiences.

Examples:

- **Biochemistry:** During an evening shift, I noticed that QC on the electrolyte analyser repeatedly failed for potassium. Troubleshooting showed that a reagent bottle was contaminated. I logged the error, recorded the corrective step (changing the reagent and recalibrating), and highlighted it for follow-up. The log later helped update the SOP to remind staff to check reagent seals carefully.

- **Haematology:** On another occasion, a clot was aspirated into the FBC analyser, leading to multiple error flags. I flushed the channels, performed maintenance, and re-ran QC. I logged the incident, including the maintenance steps, so that other staff could replicate the corrective action in similar situations.

- **Microbiology:** In urine culture, a batch of chromogenic agar plates was found to be contaminated. I stopped further use, quarantined the batch, and logged the error under "media failure," noting the batch details. This was later traced to storage issues and corrected.

- **Transfusion:** An error was identified when an analyser produced discrepant blood group results due to a calibration drift. After troubleshooting, I escalated the issue to the senior BMS and logged the event, ensuring that it was reviewed at the laboratory's incident meeting.

By logging these events, I not only contributed to immediate problem resolution but also helped the team identify patterns, improve training, and update SOPs. This process aligns with ISO15189 requirements for continual quality improvement.

Summary:

Error logging is the process of recording laboratory errors such as equipment failures, reagent issues, or procedural deviations in line with the QMS. It ensures traceability, supports corrective actions, and prevents recurrence. For example (apply as appropriate to you), logging analyser QC failures in biochemistry, clot aspiration in haematology, contaminated culture media in microbiology, or calibration drift in transfusion ensures that issues are properly documented, escalated, and used to improve practice.

Question 16:

What do you do when your LIMS goes down?

Background:

This question tests how you handle system failures that can significantly disrupt laboratory workflow. The Laboratory Information Management System (LIMS) is central to booking samples, documenting patient details, recording results, and communicating with wards. When it goes down, the risk to turnaround time (TAT) and patient safety increases, and your ability to adapt and implement contingency measures is being assessed.

Points to consider:

- What is LIMS
- Importance of LIMS in patient care and QA
- Manual documentation and communication when LIMS fail.
- Manual transfer of records into LIMS once restored
- Examples
-

Answer:

The Laboratory Information Management System (LIMS) is an electronic system used to manage patient data, book samples, record analytical results, and ensure results are easily accessible to clinicians. It also supports traceability and accountability, as all actions are logged and can be audited. Without LIMS, the laboratory faces significant disruption, particularly to sample workflow, reporting, and TAT.

When the Laboratory Information Management System (LIMS) goes down, the first step is to report the issue to IT, as a simple interface reset or server reboot can often resolve the problem quickly. If the issue persists, contingency measures are implemented to ensure that urgent testing and patient care are not compromised.

I would notify clinical areas, including wards, A&E, and theatres, of the downtime and request that only urgent or essential samples be sent until LIMS is restored. This approach helps manage the workload and prioritises patient safety.

Practical steps I would take include:

1. **Manual booking and tracking:**
   - Use laboratory request forms or downtime worksheets to manually record patient details, test requests, and sample identifiers.

   - Samples are booked directly onto the analyser where possible to avoid delays.

2. **Result recording and communication:**
   - Results generated by analysers are printed out, documented on downtime worksheets, and photocopied where needed.

   - A copy is sent to the requesting ward/department, and another copy is retained in the lab for cross-checking once LIMS is back online.

   - Urgent results (e.g., high potassium, low haemoglobin, or abnormal INR) are phoned through directly to the requesting clinician and documented manually.

3. **Storage of non-urgent samples:**
   - Where appropriate (e.g., biochemistry serum/plasma, haematology EDTA samples), non-urgent work is stored under correct temperature conditions until the system is restored. This prevents sample degradation and avoids loss of critical results.

4. **Post-restoration reconciliation:**
   - Once LIMS is restored, all manually logged data and results are entered back into the system to ensure completeness and continuity of patient records.

- Any discrepancies are reviewed and investigated to maintain data integrity.

Examples across departments (Apply as appropriate to the department you being interviewed):

- **Biochemistry:** If LIMS fails, urgent tests such as electrolytes or troponin can still be run directly on the analyser. Results are printed and phoned to A&E or cardiology teams, while documentation is kept for later upload into LIMS.

- **Haematology:** In the event of suspected sepsis, a full blood count would be prioritised, and results phoned to clinicians immediately. Coagulation results (e.g., INR for patients on warfarin) would also be fast-tracked manually.

- **Transfusion:** This is particularly critical, as patient safety is at higher risk. Paper-based systems would be used to track blood requests, issue blood units, and ensure traceability. Extra care must be taken with crossmatch records and compatibility documentation to avoid errors.

- **Microbiology:** While cultures may still be set up, results entry would be delayed. Urgent Gram stain findings, such as Gram-negative rods in a suspected meningitis case, would be phoned directly to clinicians and manually documented.

Summary

When LIMS goes down, my priority is to maintain patient safety and minimise disruption to turnaround times. The first step is to report the problem to IT and notify clinical areas (wards, A&E, theatres) so they are aware of the downtime and can prioritise sending only urgent samples.

In the lab, I switch to manual systems:

- ***Use request forms or downtime worksheets to record patient details, test requests, and sample identifiers.***

- ***Book urgent samples directly onto the analyser where possible.***

- ***Print analyser results, document them on downtime worksheets, and phone critical values (e.g., high potassium, abnormal INR, low haemoglobin, or transfusion compatibility) to the relevant ward or clinician.***

- ***Keep duplicate copies in the lab for later reconciliation.***

Non-urgent samples are stored appropriately (e.g., serum in biochemistry fridges, EDTA samples in haematology) until the system is restored. In transfusion, strict paper-based traceability is used to ensure safe issue of blood units.

Once LIMS is restored, all manually recorded information is carefully entered into the system, and any discrepancies are thoroughly investigated. This process ensures continuity of records, supports audit trails, and maintains compliance with ISO 15189 and patient safety requirements.

Question 17:

How will you resolve conflict between you and a colleague?

Background:

Pathology laboratories are complex and dynamic environments, attracting staff from different ethical, cultural, and professional backgrounds. Differences in approach or misunderstandings can arise, which, if not managed effectively, may indirectly or directly affect patient safety and laboratory service quality. This question aims to assess your ability to manage interpersonal conflict professionally while prioritising patient care.

Points consider:

- Acknowledge individual differences
- Focus on patient safety and service quality
- Use effective communication to resolve conflicts
- Escalate to senior staff or lab manager if resolution is not possible

Answer:

In a pathology laboratory, teamwork is essential to ensure patient safety, accurate results, and timely service. When a conflict arises with a colleague, I first try to understand the root cause, as many conflicts result from miscommunication or differing perspectives. I would calmly discuss the issue with the colleague, listen to their viewpoint, and clarify mine to find common ground. For example, in haematology, if there is a disagreement about prioritising urgent blood samples, I would explain my reasoning while considering their perspective to agree on a safe plan for processing.

If personal efforts do not resolve the conflict, I would escalate the matter to a senior biomedical scientist or lab manager for impartial mediation. For instance, in biochemistry, if there were repeated disagreements about who should troubleshoot a faulty analyser during a night shift, involving a senior would ensure tasks are clearly defined and patient results are not delayed.

Throughout, my focus remains on professionalism, communication, and maintaining teamwork to ensure patient care is never compromised. I am also willing to apologise if appropriate and suggest practical compromises to restore a positive working relationship.

Summary:

To resolve a conflict with a colleague, I would first identify the root cause and communicate openly to clarify any misunderstandings. I would listen actively to their perspective and share my own, seeking practical compromises while maintaining professionalism. If the conflict cannot be resolved directly, I would escalate the issue to a senior staff

member or laboratory manager to ensure an impartial resolution. Throughout the process, my focus remains on maintaining teamwork, professionalism, and prioritising patient safety and service quality.

Question 18:

Tell us your areas of strength and weakness

Background:

In a pathology laboratory, team members bring different strengths and weaknesses. Recognising your own areas of strength and weakness is important to ensure that laboratory standards are maintained in line with ISO15189, that patient safety is not compromised, and that the team functions effectively. This question assesses your self-awareness, ability to reflect, and how you manage areas of weakness to maintain quality service.

Points to consider:

- Identify key strengths and provide practical examples.
- Explain approaches to enhancing strengths.
- Identify weaknesses and explain strategies to prevent them from impacting laboratory standards.

Answer:

Over my [X years] of working in the pathology laboratory, I have identified several key areas of strength. These include my ability to work effectively in a team, multitask efficiently, stay focused under pressure, and communicate complex information clearly. For example, during busy evening shifts in haematology, I have coordinated with other colleagues to prioritise urgent samples while also validating routine samples, ensuring that turnaround times (TAT) were maintained without compromising accuracy. Similarly, in biochemistry, when an analyser requires troubleshooting while multiple samples are waiting, I have successfully balanced resolving the issue and communicating with clinicians to ensure urgent patient care needs are met.

Example 1:

Regarding weaknesses, I have noticed that I sometimes find it challenging to directly confront a colleague when I believe support is needed or when workload sharing is not optimised. For example, if a colleague has not offered assistance during a high workload period, I may initially hesitate to ask for help, attempting to complete the tasks independently. I recognise that this can affect team efficiency and potentially impact TAT.

To manage this weakness, I have developed strategies such as being proactive in communicating with my team. I make it clear when I may need assistance and encourage colleagues to offer support when they notice I am handling multiple critical tasks. Additionally, I reflect after each shift on instances where teamwork could have been optimised and plan ways to address these situations more effectively in the future. Over time, this has improved both my confidence in requesting support and my contribution to overall team cohesion and laboratory efficiency.

Example 2:

I have sometimes noticed that I can be overly meticulous when validating complex results, particularly in areas like blood transfusion or biochemistry panels with multiple parameters. While attention to detail is a strength, this can occasionally slow down the turnaround time for less urgent samples if I do not prioritise effectively.

To mitigate this, I have developed a system to prioritise urgent or critical samples while maintaining accuracy on routine tests. For example, when processing multiple biochemistry samples during a busy shift, I first check samples flagged as urgent (e.g., high potassium, critical INR, or pre-operative tests) while scheduling detailed validation of routine panels slightly later, but still within acceptable TAT limits. I also communicate with colleagues to ensure workflow is coordinated, which maintains both accuracy and efficiency

Summary:

My key strengths include teamwork, hardworking, multitasking, attention to detail, and effective communication of complex information. These qualities allow me to contribute significantly to maintaining laboratory standards, ensuring accuracy, and supporting patient care. For example, I can manage multiple urgent samples while coordinating with colleagues, ensuring TAT is met without compromising quality.

Regarding weaknesses, one area I have identified is that I sometimes find it difficult to ask for help from colleagues when workload increases or support is required. In the past, this has led me to complete tasks alone that would have been more efficiently managed with assistance. To address this, I now communicate openly with my team about when I may need support, and I proactively request help when necessary, ensuring that patient care and laboratory standards are maintained.

Another area of weakness is being overly meticulous when validating complex results, such as multi-parameter biochemistry samples or transfusion-related tests. While this attention to detail ensures accuracy, it can sometimes slow the turnaround time for routine samples. To manage this, I prioritise urgent samples, coordinate with colleagues, and schedule detailed validation for routine results within acceptable TAT limits, maintaining a balance between accuracy and efficiency.

By recognising both strengths and weaknesses and taking deliberate actions to improve or mitigate them, I ensure that my performance continues to support laboratory quality, patient safety, and team effectiveness.

Question 19:

If given this job, where do you think in the next 5 years you will be?

Background:

This question is testing whether you see yourself staying with the organisation long-term. Trusts often prefer to invest in staff who plan to remain and grow within the organisation. The aim is to gauge your ambition, commitment, and understanding of how your career path aligns with the Trust's opportunities.

Point to consider:

- Academic and qualifications background
- Current experience
- Experience to gain with the Trust
- Career progression within the Trust

Answer:

If offered this position, I see myself fully integrated into the Trust over the next five years, developing both professionally and technically.

Firstly, I plan to complete all competencies and become fully confident on the shift rota. This would allow me to manage routine and urgent samples independently while maintaining turnaround times and supporting colleagues. For example, I could manage a sudden influx of GP and ward samples in haematology or biochemistry without delaying results, ensuring patient care is not compromised.

Secondly, I aim to further my professional development, including completing a specialist portfolio (i.e if you have not already done). This would enhance my ability to handle complex tasks, such as investigating transfusion reactions in the transfusion lab or interpreting challenging coagulation and LFT results in biochemistry, contributing to accurate diagnosis and patient safety.

Thirdly, I aim to take on additional responsibilities, including participation in audits, quality control investigations, and mentoring junior staff or students. For example, leading a QC investigation or an internal audit in microbiology could help improve laboratory processes while developing my leadership skills.

Finally, I aspire to progress to more senior roles, such as Band 6 and ultimately Band 7 biomedical scientist, contributing to service improvement projects and departmental planning. For instance, I could optimise workflow in biochemistry or streamline microbiology reporting, supporting the laboratory in maintaining high-quality service in line with ISO 15189 and UKAS standards.

Overall, I see myself as a long-term member of the Trust, continuously developing my skills, supporting colleagues, and ensuring high-quality patient care while making a meaningful contribution to the success of the laboratory team.

Summary:

Over the next five years, I see myself fully integrated into the Trust, completing all competencies and confidently working on the shift rota. I aim to continue my professional development, including completing a specialist portfolio (if not already done), allowing me to handle complex tasks such as investigating transfusion reactions, interpreting challenging biochemistry results, and supporting accurate diagnosis. I also plan to take on additional responsibilities, including internal audits, quality control investigations, and mentoring junior staff. Ultimately, I aspire to progress to Band 6 and Band 7 roles, contributing to service improvement projects, departmental planning, and leadership, all while maintaining high-quality patient care and aligning my growth with the Trust's values and ISO15189 standards.

Question 20:

You are on night shift with your colleague, and you receive a call from switchboard to tell you there is an emergency. What actions would you take in order of priority?

Background:

This question tests your understanding of what constitutes an urgent or emergency situation in the laboratory, and how you respond. It also assesses your ability to multitask, delegate, communicate effectively, plan, and prioritise while ensuring laboratory standards and patient safety are maintained. Emergencies can range from urgent transfusions to critical blood test results that directly affect patient care.

Point to consider:

- Recognise and define an emergency in a clinical context.
- Communicate effectively with colleagues and clinical teams.
- Prioritise tasks to ensure urgent requests are handled first.
- Respond appropriately while maintaining accuracy and safety.

Answer:

When receiving a call about an emergency during a night shift, I would first gather all relevant information from the switchboard. This includes the patient's details, their location (ward or department), and the nature of the emergency. For example, in transfusion, it may involve providing urgent blood for a bleeding patient; in biochemistry, it could be a critically high potassium level requiring immediate attention; and in haematology, a patient may need urgent FBC or coagulation results prior to surgery.

Next, I would communicate the situation clearly with my colleague. Working together, we can divide responsibilities efficiently. For example, one person may handle the emergency sample processing while the other continues routine testing to ensure laboratory workflow is maintained. This ensures patient safety is prioritised while other tasks are not neglected.

I would then prioritise tasks based on urgency:

- For urgent blood transfusion requests, I would locate the patient's blood group, check the crossmatch history, ensure paperwork is ready, and issue compatible blood products without delay.

- For urgent critical biochemistry results, I would process the sample immediately, validate results, and communicate them to the ward promptly.

- For urgent microbiology requests (e.g., CSF for meningitis), I would ensure the sample is handled under aseptic conditions and fast-tracked for immediate analysis.

While focusing on the emergency, I would prepare for potential issues that may delay resolution. For example, ensuring all reagents are ready, analysers are functioning, and documentation is accurate so that nothing hinders patient care. Once the urgent task is completed, I would document the event, noting actions taken, communication, and outcome in the lab records or handover notes for continuity.

Summary:

In an emergency while on night shift with a colleague, I would first gather as much information as possible about the patient and the nature of the emergency to understand its urgency. I would communicate effectively with my colleague to divide tasks and manage the workload efficiently, ensuring that patient care remains the top priority. I would prioritise actions based on immediate needs, such as processing urgent samples in biochemistry, preparing compatible blood in transfusion, or handling critical microbiology specimens. I would also be proactive by ensuring all necessary resources, reagents, and documentation are ready to prevent delays. Finally, I would document all actions accurately in LIMS, lab notes, and handover sheets to maintain continuity of care and support quality assurance. This approach ensures a rapid,

safe, and effective response while upholding laboratory standards and patient safety.

Question 21:

You receive a call from the General Practice (GP) asking you for help in interpreting a result, how do you respond?

Background:

This question is testing your understanding of the scope of practice as a biomedical scientist or laboratory staff member. It assesses whether you know the limits of your role and whether you are able to communicate appropriately without overstepping into clinical decision-making, which is the responsibility of medical doctors and consultants.

Points to consider:

- Scope of practice
- Communication skills
- Referral/escalation to the appropriate professional (Consultant or Clinical Scientist)

Answer:

As a biomedical scientist, I recognise that it is important to always function strictly within my scope of practice. My role involves the analysis, validation, and reporting of laboratory results using evidence-based scientific principles, but it does not extend to giving medical advice, predicting patient outcomes, or suggesting treatment options.

If I receive a call from a GP requesting help with a result, I would first clarify exactly what they are asking. For example, if the GP needs confirmation of the reference range or whether a result falls outside normal limits, it is within my role to provide that information. I can confirm whether the result is high, low, or normal and, where relevant, direct them to existing guidelines, such as blood transfusion protocols.

However, if the GP is seeking clinical interpretation, such as what the result means for the patient's diagnosis or treatment, I would politely and clearly explain that this falls outside my scope of practice. In such cases, I would escalate appropriately by offering to transfer the call to the laboratory consultant or clinical scientist who is qualified to provide this advice.

Practical Examples:

- **Haematology:**

If a GP calls regarding a very low haemoglobin result, I can confirm that the value is significantly below the normal reference range and therefore critical. I would explain that I have already phoned the result as per SOP and note that it requires urgent clinical review. If the GP then asks whether the patient should be transfused, I will escalate to the haematology consultant, as that decision is outside my role.

- **Biochemistry:**

If a GP queries a critical potassium result, I can confirm that the result is abnormal and that, as per protocol, it has already been phoned as an urgent result. If the GP asks whether to start specific treatments (e.g., insulin-glucose infusion), I will escalate to the clinical biochemist or duty consultant.

- **Microbiology:**

If a GP asks about a positive blood culture, I can state that the organism identified is, for example, E. coli and that sensitivity testing is underway. However, if they ask which antibiotics to prescribe, I will escalate to the microbiology consultant, who is responsible for clinical decision-making.

- **Histopathology:**

If a GP calls about a biopsy result and asks what the finding means for cancer staging, I would state that the report has been issued but redirect the GP to the pathologist or consultant who can interpret the result in clinical context.

Summary:

If a GP calls requesting help with a result, I can confirm whether it is normal, high, or low and direct them to relevant guidelines. However, I do not provide clinical advice or suggest treatment, as this is beyond my scope of practice. In such cases, I would politely explain this and escalate the query to the appropriate consultant or clinical scientist, such as a haematology consultant for blood results, a clinical biochemist for biochemical tests, or a microbiology consultant for culture results.

Question 22:

How do you demonstrate our trust values in your place of work? Compassion, courage, integrity, accountability, respect. Which of them is most important to you?

Background:

This question is three in one. It is testing how your professional ethics align with the Trust's values, how you practically demonstrate each of these values, and finally, which value is most important to you (with examples). You should avoid generic answers by tying each value to real-life situations in the lab, showing how they influence your daily practice and patient care.

Point to consider:

- Identify and reflect on the Trust values.
- Connect them with your professional ethics as a biomedical scientist.
- Use practical laboratory examples to show how you live out these values.
- Clearly explain which value resonates most with you and why.

Answer:

I am very motivated by this position, partly because the Trust values, which are compassion, courage, integrity, accountability, and respect resonate strongly with my professional and personal ethics. Each value is key in ensuring patient safety and maintaining the high standards expected in an ISO15189 accredited laboratory. I will demonstrate how I apply each in my daily work.

- **Compassion:** I always remember that every sample represents a real patient, often anxious or unwell. For example, in haematology, when handling urgent full blood counts for patients suspected of sepsis, I ensure these are processed immediately, even when the workload is heavy. Treating every sample as if it belonged to me or my family helps me focus on patient wellbeing beyond just numbers on a screen.

- **Courage:** In the lab, courage is often about speaking up and making difficult decisions under pressure. For example, during a biochemistry night shift, I once had to question and reject a batch of patient results because QC had failed. Although it delayed release, I had the courage to escalate the issue to the duty biochemist rather than risk releasing potentially misleading results. This demonstrated putting patient safety before convenience.

- **Integrity:** Mistakes can happen in a busy lab, but integrity means being honest and transparent. For example, in microbiology, if I notice an error in sample labelling during culture processing, I stop the process and raise a non-conformance report, even if it delays the workflow. I believe hiding mistakes would compromise trust, whereas integrity helps maintain patient safety and professional standards.

- **Accountability:** I take responsibility for my work and follow through on my duties. For instance, in blood transfusion, if I issue blood products during an emergency, I always ensure the full traceability paperwork is completed and checked before and after issue, even under pressure. This accountability ensures compliance with MHRA requirements and helps avoid risks to patient safety.

- **Respect:** The pathology lab brings together people of diverse backgrounds and expertise. Respect is essential for teamwork. For example, when lone working in histopathology specimen reception with a new MLA, I took the time to explain procedures respectfully, acknowledging their learning pace, rather than rushing them. This built trust, improved efficiency, and ensured we maintained accuracy.

Of all these values, the one that resonates most strongly with me is integrity. Without integrity, other values lose their strength: compassion without honesty can mislead, courage without transparency can harm, and accountability without truth is incomplete. A good example was when I once validated abnormal coagulation results that could not be explained clinically. Rather than releasing them, I stopped, repeated the test, and escalated to the senior scientist. The results were indeed erroneous, and by acting with integrity, I prevented potential mismanagement of the patient.

Summary:

I demonstrate the Trust values in my daily work by: showing compassion by treating every sample as a patient; courage by escalating issues or rejecting results when patient safety is at risk; integrity by being honest and transparent about mistakes; accountability by taking responsibility for my work, particularly in regulated areas like blood transfusion; and respect by working collaboratively and valuing colleagues. The value most important to me is integrity, because it underpins trust, professionalism, and patient safety in everything I do.

Question 23:

What value will you bring to the team?

Background:

Job adverts are usually posted because there is a specific need within the team. This question tests whether you can bring qualities, experiences, or skills that not only meet the essential and desirable criteria in the person specification but also complement and strengthen the existing team. Concentrating on your technical expertise, transferable skills, and alignment with Trust values is the best approach.

Points to consider:

- Study the person specification carefully.
- Highlight your relevant experience and skills.
- Use practical examples that connect to laboratory work.
- Demonstrate how your contribution supports patient care and the wider team.

Answer:

I am passionate about this position, and I believe that both my academic qualifications and professional experiences have prepared me to add real value to the team.

Firstly, I bring strong technical competence across core laboratory disciplines. In haematology, for example, I am confident in validating complex blood count results, recognising critical values such as blasts in leukaemia or severe anaemia, and escalating appropriately. In biochemistry, I have experience troubleshooting analyser errors, including blocked probes or failed calibrations, documenting root causes, and implementing corrective actions. In blood transfusion, I am competent in antibody screening and issuing blood in emergency situations while ensuring full traceability. These technical skills enable me to contribute effectively to service delivery from day one.

Secondly, I bring problem-solving and troubleshooting skills, which are vital in a busy 24/7 lab. For example, during a weekend shift in biochemistry, when one analyser went down, I quickly isolated it, diverted samples to the backup analyser, and worked with IT to resolve the interface error. This proactive approach minimised turnaround time for urgent A&E samples. Such experiences show that I can remain calm under pressure and support patient care by prioritising effectively.

Beyond technical expertise, I also bring transferable skills that strengthen the team:

- **Teamwork and communication:** I work collaboratively with colleagues, whether that is sharing workload during peak demand or handing over complex cases clearly to the next shift. For instance, in microbiology, when we had a backlog of urine cultures, I coordinated with colleagues to divide tasks efficiently, which helped us clear the pending cases without compromising quality.

- **Training and mentoring:** I enjoy supporting junior colleagues. In my previous role, I assisted new trainees in learning analyser maintenance procedures, which sped up their competency sign-off and improved rota flexibility.

- **IT and digital skills:** With increasing reliance on LIMS and middleware systems, my ability to navigate these systems effectively and even support colleagues with troubleshooting helps ensure smooth operation.

Finally, I bring a strong alignment with the Trust values (**assuming the values are accountability, integrity, and respect**). For example, I show accountability by ensuring all non-conformances are properly logged and investigated; integrity by being transparent about errors; and respect by valuing the contributions of colleagues across disciplines, from MLAs to senior scientists. I believe these values will allow me to fit seamlessly into the team culture and contribute to continuous improvement in line with ISO15189.

Summary:

The value I will bring to the team includes strong technical competence across haematology, biochemistry, transfusion, and microbiology, alongside effective troubleshooting and problem-solving skills. I also offer transferable strengths in teamwork, communication, training, and IT. In addition, I am aligned with the Trust's values, ensuring that my contribution supports high-quality patient care while enhancing the overall performance and resilience of the laboratory team.

Question 24:

What is Audit and how do you participate in audit?

Background:

This question is testing your knowledge of laboratory audit within the framework of Quality Management Systems (QMS) and Quality Assurance (QA). An audit checks whether the laboratory is working in line with ISO15189 standards and the requirements of regulatory bodies such as UKAS. The panel also wants to know if you understand the different types of audits (internal and external) and the role that every staff member plays in preparing for and participating in audits.

Point to consider:

- Define audit clearly.
- Show awareness of internal and external audits.
- Mention audit types (vertical, horizontal, witness/examination, clinical).
- Highlight staff responsibilities in preparation and participation.
- Give practical examples from your own lab experiences.

Answer:

An audit is a structured process within the Quality Management System (QMS) that assesses whether a laboratory is adhering to established standards and procedures. In the UK, external audits are conducted by UKAS to ensure compliance with ISO15189 requirements. Internal audits are performed by laboratory staff to monitor compliance and identify areas for improvement before external assessment. Together, these audits are central to maintaining quality assurance and patient safety.

There are different types of audits:

- **Vertical audit:** following a single sample from request to reporting, ensuring all steps are compliant.

- **Horizontal audit:** looking at one process across multiple areas, e.g., analyser maintenance records.

- **Witness/examination audit:** observing a member of staff carrying out a procedure, such as analyser calibration.

- **Clinical audit:** assessing the appropriateness of tests ordered or the impact of results on patient care.

To prepare for an audit, laboratories ensure that all documentation and records are up to date. This includes training and competency signoffs, analyser maintenance logs (daily, weekly, monthly), IQC and EQA records, stock management, incident logs, and SOPs. Staff also play a role in ensuring the physical laboratory environment such as cleanliness, labelling, and safety checks meets standards.

In terms of my participation, I have supported audits in several ways (Use where appropriate to you):

- **In haematology,** I helped review analyser maintenance records. When I noticed missing daily checks, I escalated this to my senior so it could be corrected before the audit.

- **In biochemistry,** I contributed by checking IQC documentation, ensuring that corrective actions for out-of-range controls were fully recorded.

- **In blood transfusion,** I supported preparation by checking fridge temperature records and expiry date monitoring of blood units, both of which are critical for traceability.

- **During one external UKAS visit,** I was nominated to speak with the auditor about result validation in haematology. I explained how I validate results against reference ranges, flag critical results, and escalate abnormalities appropriately. The auditor was satisfied with my explanation and documentation, which reflected positively on the department.

- I also ensure that my training and competency records are always up to date, as auditors may ask staff to provide evidence of their qualifications and competencies. In one internal audit, I was observed performing a daily analyser quality control check. By clearly explaining each step and referencing the relevant SOP, I was able to demonstrate both compliance and understanding, contributing to a successful audit outcome.

Overall, my approach to audit participation is to be thorough, proactive, and accountable, ensuring that both my individual work and the department as a whole meet the required standards.

Summary:

An audit is a QMS tool that checks laboratory compliance with ISO15189 standards. Audit assessment can be carried out internally by staff and externally by UKAS. There are different types: vertical, horizontal, witness, and clinical. My role in audits includes keeping my training and competency records up to date, reviewing QC and analyser maintenance logs, checking blood product traceability, and ensuring SOPs are followed. I have also spoken directly with auditors about result validation, which reflected positively on my work and the department. Through these contributions, I help maintain quality assurance and continuous improvement in line with patient safety and Trust standards.

Question 25:

What is Batch testing?

Background:

This question is testing your understanding of the process of testing laboratory materials (e.g., reagents, kits, consumables) before they are introduced into routine use. It is an essential part of the laboratory Quality Management System (QMS) and helps ensure results are reliable, reproducible, and consistent with the manufacturer's claims. Batch testing is also closely tied to ISO15189 requirements, as it forms part of quality assurance and risk minimisation in patient testing.

Points to consider:

- What is batch testing
- Reason for batch testing
- Connect to ISO15189 requirements.

Answer:

Batch testing is a quality control process performed in the laboratory to check the suitability of new reagents, kits, or other consumables before they are put into routine use. Every time a new batch or lot number is received, it must be tested against known control samples (positive, negative, or normal ranges depending on the test). This ensures that the product gives results consistent with the manufacturer's specifications and with the laboratory's expected performance.

The same principle applies if a reagent is approaching the end of its use or if a change in formulation, storage, or supplier occurs. This helps the laboratory maintain traceability, accuracy, and reproducibility, as required under ISO15189.

Reasons for batch testing include:

- To verify reliability and accuracy of new materials.

- To detect manufacturing defects or degradation that could compromise results.

- To maintain patient safety by ensuring all materials used meet quality standards.

- To comply with ISO15189 and UKAS requirements on quality assurance and equipment validation.

Practical Examples across Laboratory Departments:

- **Haematology:**

When receiving a new batch of reagents for the full blood count analyser, batch testing is performed by running internal QC material and comparing results with previous batch performance. For specific assays, such as Infectious Mononucleosis (IM) kits, known positive and negative samples are used. If the new batch gives expected results, it is validated for use.

- **Biochemistry:**

When a new lot of glucose reagent is delivered, the laboratory tests it by running internal QC material and patient samples with known results. The new batch is only approved if values align with expected ranges and correlate well with the previous batch, ensuring no drift in patient results.

- **Microbiology:**

If a new batch of antibiotic susceptibility discs arrives, batch testing is carried out by using control organisms (e.g., E. coli ATCC 25922). Zone diameters must fall within specified ranges provided by EUCAST/CLSI guidelines. This validates the discs before they are used on patient isolates.

- **Transfusion (Blood Bank):**

When a new lot of antibody screening cells is received, they are batch tested against known control plasma samples to confirm that expected antibodies are detected. This ensures no false negatives/positives occur when screening patient samples for transfusion compatibility.

- **Histology:**

For a new batch of special stains (e.g., PAS or Gram stains), known tissue control slides are used. The stain is only accepted if it demonstrates the expected staining pattern, ensuring diagnostic reliability in routine use.

Summary:

Batch testing is the process of checking new laboratory reagents, kits, or consumables against known controls to ensure they produce accurate and reliable results before use in patient testing. It is carried out in all departments (e.g., reagent checks in biochemistry, antibiotic disc checks in microbiology, antibody cell screening in transfusion, or stain validation in histology). The main purpose is to confirm manufacturer claims, maintain patient safety, and comply with ISO15189 standards.

Question 26:

When have you felt overwhelmed and how did you deal with it?

Background:

Pathology laboratories are highly complex and often pressured environments. Emergencies, unexpected workload surges, short staffing, or equipment breakdowns can easily create overwhelming situations. The purpose of this question is to test your ability to maintain composure, prioritise effectively, seek help where necessary, and ensure laboratory standards and patient safety are not compromised.

Points to consider:

- Give a real example of when you felt overwhelmed.
- Show how you prioritised, planned, and sought support.

- Demonstrate that patient safety and standards were never compromised.

Answer:

There have been several occasions in the laboratory where I have felt overwhelmed, usually when multiple unexpected challenges occurred at the same time. While such situations can be unavoidable, I have learned to maintain composure, apply planning and prioritisation skills, and ask for help when required to keep the laboratory functioning safely and efficiently.

For example, during a late shift **in Haematology,** one of the main analysers broke down while I had several urgent samples pending. While troubleshooting, the backup analyser also failed, and the bench quickly became crowded with unprocessed samples. Initially, it felt overwhelming as both machines were unavailable. To regain control:

- I immediately phoned the wards to explain the situation and requested that only urgent samples be sent until further notice.

- I prioritised emergency and ward-critical samples, processing them manually to ensure patient care was not delayed.

- I separated GP and routine samples, storing them at the correct temperature until alternative arrangements could be made.

- I logged the analyser breakdown and contacted the engineer for urgent repair.

- I coordinated with another NHS site to transfer critical samples, ensuring results were phoned back for continuity of care.

Although stressful, maintaining communication and focusing on patient safety helped me manage the situation effectively.

In biochemistry, I once faced significant pressure when quality control (QC) samples repeatedly failed on an analyser. After extensive troubleshooting and recalibration, it became clear that the issue was caused by contaminated reconstituted reagents. Despite the resulting backlog and stress, I remained calm, followed the SOPs, documented the incident, and worked with a senior colleague to prepare new reagents. Once QC was successfully completed, testing resumed, and I ensured all results were properly validated to eliminate any risk to patients.

In Microbiology, an overwhelming moment occurred during a night shift when a large number of blood cultures flagged positive simultaneously, in addition to urgent CSF samples. To manage this:

- I triaged the most critical samples (CSFs first, due to possible meningitis).
- Communicated with clinicians about expected delays.
- Used my colleague's support to divide the workload. For example, one focusing on blood cultures, the other on urgent direct microscopy.

In Blood Transfusion, I have experienced overwhelming moments during a major haemorrhage call, where multiple units of blood products were required quickly. While the workload spiked and the pressure was intense, I followed the major haemorrhage protocol, worked closely with my colleague to crossmatch, and ensured products were issued in the right order. Clear communication with the clinical team ensured that the patient received timely support.

In all these cases, what helped me cope with overwhelming situations was:

- **Prioritisation:** focusing first on life-threatening or emergency cases.
- **Communication:** keeping clinicians, colleagues, and seniors informed.

- **Teamwork:** delegating and seeking support where needed.
- **Professionalism:** ensuring that even under pressure, ISO15189 standards were maintained, and all incidents were documented.

Summary:

I have felt overwhelmed in the laboratory during events such as analyser breakdowns, repeated QC failures, major haemorrhage calls, or sudden surges in urgent samples. In these situations, I stayed calm, prioritised urgent cases, communicated with colleagues and clinicians, and sought support when needed. For example, when both haematology analysers failed on a late shift, I processed urgent samples manually, stored non-urgent ones appropriately, arranged transfer to another NHS site, and informed wards to reduce sample load. In another case, when QC failed due to contaminated reagents, I reconstituted fresh reagents, recalibrated the analyser, and resumed testing. Across departments, I manage overwhelming moments by maintaining focus on patient safety, clear communication, and adherence to SOPs, ensuring that standards are never compromised.

Question 27:

How do you concentrate in a noisy environment?

Background:

Noise is sometimes unavoidable in the laboratory, whether from analysers, telephones, emergency calls, or even colleagues discussing work-related matters. Excessive noise can increase the risk of distraction, mistakes, and stress, which can directly or indirectly impact patient safety and the overall laboratory quality. This question tests your ability to maintain focus, use practical strategies to limit distractions, and ensure standards are not compromised.

Points to consider:

- Recognise that noise is part of the lab environment.
- Show strategies you use to remain focused.
- Provide practical examples of how you managed noise without compromising standards.

Answer:

I recognise that noise is an inherent part of the laboratory environment and cannot always be avoided, but patient safety must never be compromised. To manage this effectively, I use a combination of proactive and reactive strategies.

For example, if noise arises from colleagues' non-work-related conversations and disrupts my focus, I politely ask them to lower their voices. If the issue persists and significantly affects my concentration, I escalate it to a senior member of staff so that it can be addressed professionally.

In situations where noise cannot be controlled, such as from analysers running, alarms sounding, or multiple phone calls, I increase my focus by prioritising tasks, maintaining clear organisation, and using checklists to ensure that all procedures are followed accurately, thereby safeguarding both patient safety and the quality of laboratory work.

- Double-checking every entry or result validation before confirming.

- Reading back details (patient name, date of birth, hospital number) aloud quietly to myself to ensure accuracy.

- Breaking complex tasks into smaller steps so I do not lose track in the middle of distractions.

- If unsure, asking a senior colleague to verify my work before finalising.

Practical examples:

- **In Haematology,** during a busy shift when analysers were beeping frequently for QC and flags, I had to validate a critical neutropenic result. Despite the noisy background, I carefully read the result against the patient's previous history on LIMS, validated it, and phoned it immediately to the ward without error.

- **In Biochemistry,** when multiple phones were ringing at once and the lab was short-staffed, I was booking samples. To maintain accuracy, I slowed down slightly, repeated patient identifiers aloud, and cross-checked them against request forms before processing.

- **In Microbiology,** I was preparing microscopy slides when the blood culture analyser flagged multiple positive bottles at once and the phones were ringing continuously with wards chasing urgent results. To stay focused, I documented each slide preparation step clearly and set aside urgent culture bottles in a separate tray to process systematically. I also asked a colleague to temporarily handle phone queries so I could finish the microscopy without error, then double-checked my findings before reporting.

- **In Blood Transfusion,** during a busy evening with constant phone calls for blood products, I ensured concentration by following the "read back" process, checking every unit number and patient detail twice before issuing, even if phones kept ringing. This prevented issuing errors.

Overall, my approach is to control what I can (like unnecessary conversations), and for noise that I cannot control, I increase my concentration by slowing down, double-checking, and asking for verification when needed. This ensures that even in a noisy environment, accuracy and patient safety are not compromised.

Summary:

I manage noisy environments by controlling what I can, such as politely asking colleagues to lower their voices, and by maintaining focus when noise is unavoidable, for example from analysers or phones. I achieve this by double-checking results, reading patient details aloud to myself, breaking tasks into smaller steps, and seeking verification if uncertain. For instance, in blood transfusion during a noisy evening with multiple phone calls, I carefully followed the "read back" process to ensure the correct blood products were issued. Similarly, in haematology and biochemistry, I validated results and processed samples accurately despite analyser alarms and phone interruptions by slowing down and rechecking each step. These strategies enable me to remain focused, accurate, and patient-centred even in challenging, noisy environments.

Question 28:

Tell us about a time you dealt with a difficult colleague

Background:

As mentioned previously, the complex and dynamic nature of pathology laboratories attracts staff from different professional, ethical, and cultural backgrounds. While this diversity enriches the team, it can sometimes lead to misunderstandings or conflicts. This question is testing your ability to recognise such challenges and manage them in a way that does not compromise laboratory standards, turnaround times (TAT), or, most importantly, patient safety.

Points to consider:

- The diverse nature of the laboratory environment.
- Differences among staff and how they can cause friction.
- Always keeping the patient as the priority.
- Using effective communication and escalation where necessary.
- Practical examples of how you resolved such situations.

Answer:

In a busy laboratory environment, differences between colleagues are not unusual. These can arise from personal backgrounds, working styles, or the stress of a high workload. What matters most is ensuring that such differences never affect patient care or laboratory standards. For my part, I always aim to communicate professionally, remain calm, and keep every action focused on the wellbeing of the patient.

For example, **in haematology,** I once worked with a colleague during a busy night shift where there was a disagreement about prioritising urgent samples. They wanted to process GP samples immediately, but I reminded them that A&E and maternity ward samples had to come first, as per our SOP. I explained my reasoning politely, referred to the guidelines, and we agreed on a clear plan. By keeping the discussion centred on patient safety, we avoided conflict and ensured timely results for urgent patients.

In biochemistry, I experienced a situation where a colleague became visibly frustrated after repeated QC failures on an analyser. Their frustration began to affect communication, which could have delayed urgent samples. To ease the pressure, I offered to take over loading routine samples while they focused on troubleshooting. This kept the workflow moving and gave them space to resolve the issue calmly.

In microbiology, I worked alongside a colleague who was reluctant to share key observations about a culture plate, insisting it was "not their responsibility." Knowing this could delay reporting, I encouraged them by explaining how sharing their findings supports accuracy and patient safety. When the reluctance persisted, I escalated to the senior biomedical scientist, ensuring the issue was handled without conflict while still protecting the patient's interests.

Whenever such situations arise, my focus remains on professionalism, teamwork, and patient care. If direct communication does not resolve the issue, I escalate it to a senior colleague or manager, as allowing conflict to continue could affect the entire service.

Summary:

Dealing with difficult colleagues is part of working in a busy and diverse laboratory, but I always focus on patient care and laboratory standards. I manage such situations by communicating respectfully, staying professional, and keeping discussions centred on patient safety. For example, when a colleague disagreed with prioritising urgent samples, I calmly explained the SOPs and guided us to a solution without conflict. If direct communication is not effective, I escalate to senior staff to ensure that the service is not disrupted. This approach ensures that personal differences never compromise patient safety or laboratory quality.

Question 29:

Patient phoned in for result, what would you do? Will you give out the result?

Background:

It is not uncommon for patients to phone the laboratory directly asking for their results. This often happens when they are unable to get through to their GP or feel there are delays in communication. While patients do have a right to access their results, it is not within the scope of practice of a biomedical scientist or pathology staff to provide results directly to a patient. This is because results must always be explained in a clinical context by the responsible healthcare professional, such as the GP or hospital consultant. This question is testing whether you understand your professional boundaries, NHS guidelines, and how to communicate effectively with patients while maintaining standards.

Points to consider:

- Professional boundaries (scope of practice).
- NHS guidelines and patient confidentiality.

- Communication skills like how to reassure a potentially frustrated patient without crossing professional boundaries.

Answer:

If a patient phones the laboratory directly requesting their results, I will not give the results out, as this is outside my scope of practice and against NHS guidelines. The role of a biomedical scientist is to analyse, validate, and release results to the appropriate clinician, not to discuss results directly with patients.

My first step would be to remain calm and polite, acknowledging the patient's concern. Often, patients who phone the lab may be anxious, frustrated, or even upset after waiting for their results. I would reassure them that I understand their concern, but I would explain clearly that results can only be issued and discussed through their clinician. This ensures that confidentiality is protected and that patients receive their results in the correct context, along with the appropriate advice.

For example, in haematology, a patient may phone chasing their full blood count result. While I could technically see the result on the LIMS, I cannot disclose it. Instead, I would explain: "I'm sorry, but laboratory staff cannot issue results directly to patients. Please contact your GP or consultant, who will have access to the report and can explain what the result means for your care."

In biochemistry, patients sometimes chase tests like thyroid function or HbA1c. Again, while I may know whether a result is abnormal or not, it is not my role to explain this, as interpretation depends on the clinical picture (e.g., symptoms, treatment history). I would redirect them back to their GP or hospital consultant.

In microbiology, I have seen patients chasing swab or urine culture results. These are particularly sensitive, as they often involve infection status and antibiotic sensitivities. Giving these results directly without medical explanation could cause distress or lead to inappropriate self-medication. In such cases, I would firmly but politely advise them to contact their GP.

In blood transfusion, a patient may enquire about antibody screen results or crossmatch availability. This is especially sensitive and must only be communicated through the clinical team. In this case, I would explain the same principle and, if necessary, direct the call to the hospital switchboard so they can be connected with the appropriate clinical team.

If the patient insists or becomes distressed, I would escalate the situation by informing my senior, or advise the patient to contact the hospital's Patient Advice and Liaison Service (PALS), who are trained to support patients in accessing their records appropriately.

Summary:

If a patient phoned for their result, I would not give it out, as this is outside my scope of practice and against NHS guidelines. Instead, I would remain polite and professional, explaining that results can only be given by their GP or hospital clinician who can interpret them in context.

For example, if a patient called to chase a full blood count or a microbiology culture result, I would reassure them but redirect them to their clinician, ensuring confidentiality and patient safety. If the patient became distressed, I would escalate the situation to a senior or advise them to contact PALS. This approach allows me to maintain professionalism, protect confidentiality, and uphold laboratory standards while still showing empathy to the patient.

Question 30:

On Stress tolerance - Can you tell me about a situation where the stress you experienced made it difficult for you to complete an important task and how did you overcome this?

Background:

Pathology laboratories can be high-pressure environments due to workload, emergencies, staff shortages, and equipment issues.

This question aims to assess your ability to manage stress without compromising patient care or laboratory standards. It tests your resilience, problem-solving, and use of available support systems while ensuring compliance with ISO15189 and hospital policies.

Points to consider:

- Acknowledge possible laboratory stress
- Managing stress using established support systems within the hospital
- Maintaining focus on patient care despite stress
- Practical examples of stress management

Answer:

Stress is a common challenge in pathology laboratories, especially during periods of high workload, staff shortages, or technical problems. I have encountered situations where stress made it difficult to maintain my usual pace and focus, but I have always found strategies to manage it while keeping patient care and laboratory standards intact.

For example, there was a period when several staff members were on sick leave or had resigned. This led to short staffing, which coincided with repeated analyser breakdowns over a two-week period. During this time, I was responsible for troubleshooting the analysers while also maintaining routine sample processing and validating urgent results. The combination of technical issues and increased workload created a significant amount of stress, making it challenging to complete tasks with my usual efficiency.

To manage the situation, I took several practical steps:

1. **Communication and support:** I discussed the situation openly with my line manager, highlighting both workload and equipment issues. This allowed us to prioritise urgent tasks and plan temporary support, such as reallocating certain samples to another site or requesting additional staff to cover critical periods.

2. **Using wellbeing resources:** I utilised the hospital wellbeing department to manage the emotional impact of the stress. This included guidance on taking structured breaks and strategies for mental resilience.

3. **Task prioritisation:** I organised tasks based on urgency, for example, ensuring urgent ward or GP samples were processed first, while less critical samples were temporarily stored under appropriate conditions.

4. **Stepwise troubleshooting:** When analysers failed, I documented each troubleshooting step carefully and used previous error logs to speed up resolution. This prevented repeated mistakes and reduced stress related to uncertainty.

5. **Temporary rest:** I arranged a short period of leave to recover from burnout. Returning refreshed allowed me to resume work with renewed focus and energy.

Since that experience, I have developed stronger coping strategies for stressful situations, such as proactively managing workload, asking for support early, and ensuring structured breaks during long or demanding shifts.

For example, in biochemistry, when multiple analysers fail at the same time, I now immediately prioritise critical tests such as electrolytes and cardiac markers, while delegating non-urgent work. This helps maintain turnaround times and ensures patient safety. Similarly, in blood transfusion, if urgent crossmatch requests arrive during a period of high workload, I focus first on preparing blood products for emergency transfusions, while documenting other requests for processing as soon as it is safe to do so.

These approaches ensure that stress does not impact my technical judgment, analytical skills, or patient care, and they demonstrate my ability to remain resilient and professional under pressure.

Summary:

Stress in pathology laboratories can arise from staff shortages, equipment failure, or high workload. I manage it by communicating with line managers, using hospital wellbeing resources, prioritising urgent tasks, documenting troubleshooting steps, and taking structured breaks when needed. This approach ensures patient care and laboratory standards are maintained. Over time, I have developed practical strategies to remain resilient, organised, and focused under pressure, demonstrating effective stress tolerance in the lab environment.

Question 31:

What will you do if a GP calls you that you should process an urgent sample?

Background:

While urgent requests are common from wards and A&E, GPs sometimes phone the laboratory when they are concerned about a patient and need rapid results to decide on referral. This question tests your ability to prioritise urgent samples, communicate clearly, respect professional boundaries, and keep patient safety central.

Points to consider:

- What constitutes an urgent request and who decides it (clinician).
- Planning and prioritising workflow to fast-track urgent samples.
- Practical steps to trace, process, validate and communicate urgent results.
- When to escalate to consultants or clinical scientists.

- Documentation and adherence to ISO15189/NHS guidance.

Answer:

If a GP phones asking that a sample be processed urgently, I accept the GP's clinical judgement and act to support it. I first take full patient identifiers and the caller's details, then check whether the specimen has already arrived. If it has, I trace it and prioritise it for immediate processing; if not, I advise the GP to label it urgent and notify specimen reception so it will be flagged on arrival. I process the sample promptly, check for any pre-analytical or analytical issues, validate the result as soon as it is reliable, and then phone the GP to confirm they have received and understood the result. If the result is critical or needs specialist interpretation, I escalate immediately to the relevant consultant or clinical scientist and document the communication in line with lab policy.

Practical examples across departments:

Haematology: A GP once phoned requesting an urgent full blood count for a child with bruising and lethargy. When the sample arrived, I prioritised it immediately, ran the FBC, and validated the result, which showed a very high blast count. I phoned the GP straight away and escalated the case to the haematology consultant so the child could be admitted urgently. I also documented each step clearly in the LIMS and in the handover notes.

Biochemistry: A GP called asking for an urgent U&E for a patient with weakness and palpitations. On processing, the potassium was critically raised (hyperkalaemia). I validated the result, telephoned the GP to highlight the life-threatening value, and advised that the patient should be referred urgently; I also informed the on-call clinical biochemist for confirmation and documentation.

Microbiology: For a GP-sent CSF sample suspected of meningitis, I prioritised Gram stain and microscopy ahead of routine work, performed the tests immediately, and phoned preliminary findings to the GP (and the receiving hospital team) so clinical management could be fast-tracked while culture continued.

Transfusion: Although less frequent from GP calls, I once had a GP flag severe anaemia prior to transfer. I prioritised group & save and crossmatch, ensured blood products were prepared, and liaised with the transfusion consultant and receiving site to make sure compatible units would be available on arrival.

Summary:

If a GP requests an urgent sample, I record the patient and caller details, confirm whether the sample has been received and flag it for immediate processing, validate the result once verified, phone the GP to ensure they have the result and understand it, and escalate to the appropriate consultant when specialist input is required. I always document the actions taken. By following this approach, I support safe, timely patient care while maintaining laboratory standards and clear communication with clinical teams.

Question 32:

How do you manage other activities with your circular work?

Background:

It can be wrongly assumed that pathology laboratory work is solely about biological sample reception, booking, analysis, and releasing or validating results to support the management of patient wellbeing. While these activities are central, there are other equally important responsibilities such as competency training, internal and external audits, UKAS inspections, NEQAS participation, attending professional conferences, and engaging in continuous professional development (CPD). This question is testing your ability to balance all of these activities without compromising your core laboratory duties, which are critical for patient safety and wellbeing.

Points to consider:

- Planning and Prioritising activities
- Ensuring patient care and service delivery remain central
- Time management strategies for balancing routine work with additional responsibilities

Answer:

I manage other activities alongside my core laboratory duties by careful planning and prioritising, always ensuring that patient safety and diagnostic service delivery remain central. My approach involves assessing which activities are urgent and essential at a given time and adjusting my focus accordingly.

For example, I plan my week in advance and align my tasks with my rota to make sure I stay organised. During busy day shifts, I prioritise core duties such as sample processing and result validation, as patient demand is highest at these times. Tasks like updating my training portfolio or reviewing audit checklists are reserved for quieter weekend or night shifts, where I can complete them without impacting urgent sample turnaround times.

Example:

In haematology, I have managed this balance by ensuring my analyser maintenance and daily QC are prioritised during the day, while leaving competency documentation updates or reviewing IQC/NEQAS reports to periods of reduced workload. This allows me to remain compliant with ISO15189 requirements without compromising patient results.

In biochemistry, I recall a situation where UKAS inspectors were scheduled to review reagent lot validation records. To prepare, I worked with colleagues to ensure that batch testing documentation was completed and filed during quieter shifts, so that routine sample turnaround was not affected. By coordinating responsibilities and sharing tasks, we ensured the department was fully prepared for inspection without impacting urgent biochemistry reporting.

In microbiology, I have balanced workload by prioritising urgent samples such as CSF and blood cultures first, while allocating time during night shifts to review audit trails, update SOPs, or cross-check equipment calibration logs. This ensures both immediate patient care and long-term quality assurance are maintained.

In blood transfusion, I experienced a situation where a major haemorrhage protocol coincided with an external NEQAS assessment deadline. In that case, I prioritised patient safety by managing the urgent transfusion first, but later in the shift ensured that NEQAS results were uploaded and documented correctly, with support from my colleague. This demonstrated the importance of teamwork, flexibility, and time management in meeting multiple responsibilities.

Summary:

Managing other activities alongside core laboratory duties requires planning, prioritisation, and flexibility. I ensure that patient-focused tasks such as sample analysis and result validation always take priority, while activities like training updates, audits, and quality assurance work are scheduled during quieter periods or non-peak shifts. By staying organised and proactive, I'm able to meet the demands of routine laboratory work alongside my professional responsibilities without compromising standards or patient care.

Question 33:

Tell us about your experience and why you applied to our Trust.

Background:

This question is testing how well you align with the job description and person specification. It requires you to highlight your academic qualifications, professional experiences, areas of competency, and key skills, while also demonstrating how your personal and professional values connect with the Trust values. In addition, you are expected to show genuine interest in the Trust itself for example, whether that be its specialties, services, reputation, or location and explain how working there would support your career progression and contribution to patient care.

Points to consider:

- Passion and qualification
- Experience and areas of competency
- Skills relevant to the role
- Personal values aligned with Trust values
- Interest in the Trust's specialties, services, and location

Answer:

I have always been passionate about pursuing a career in pathology and this motivated me to study biomedical science and gain HCPC registration as a biomedical scientist. Since then, I have built up extensive experience working in different areas of the laboratory, where I have developed strong technical and professional competencies.

Example:

In haematology, I have become confident in analyser troubleshooting, including routine maintenance, calibration, and corrective actions when QC has failed. For instance, I have interpreted QC using Levey-Jennings charts and Westgard rules, identified patterns of drift, and taken appropriate actions to ensure accuracy of patient results.

In biochemistry, I have been responsible for reagent verification and validation of new batches prior to use. This often involved performing batch testing against known control samples and documenting the findings to comply with ISO15189 and UKAS requirements. I have also participated in NEQAS, reviewing external quality assessments and implementing corrective measures when performance trends highlighted the need

In microbiology, I have been competent in processing samples, preparing microscopy slides, and using culture techniques to support clinicians with timely and accurate diagnoses. For example, when working during a busy on-call period, I prioritised urgent CSF and blood culture samples, while ensuring documentation and audit trails were maintained.

In blood transfusion, I have worked within the requirements of major haemorrhage protocols, handling urgent crossmatches, and ensuring appropriate communication with clinical teams during critical incidents. This experience has taught me the importance of teamwork, accuracy, and rapid response under pressure.

Beyond my technical experience, I have developed key transferable skills such as effective communication, IT proficiency, multitasking, and teamwork. For example, I have delivered training to junior staff and supported colleagues during audits by preparing documentation and clearly demonstrating compliance procedures to inspectors.

What attracted me to this Trust in particular is how its values, which are compassion, courage, integrity, accountability, and respect. These values align closely with my own professional ethos. I strongly believe that every sample represents a patient, and so compassion and accountability guide every decision I make in the laboratory. I was also drawn to the Trust's specialty areas, particularly in [e.g., women's and children's health, trauma, or other specific services relevant to the Trust], because they represent opportunities where laboratory support is critical to patient outcomes.

I applied because I want to contribute my skills, experience, and values to a Trust that not only delivers high-quality patient care but also invests in staff development. I am confident that working here will allow me to continue to grow professionally, gain further specialist expertise, and contribute meaningfully to the Trust's mission.

Summary:

My academic background, professional experiences across multiple laboratory departments, and strong technical and interpersonal skills have equipped me to contribute effectively as a biomedical scientist in your Trust.

I am particularly motivated by how closely my professional values align with your Trust values, and by the Trust's strong commitment to patient-centred care, especially in women and children's health and trauma services. I believe I can contribute meaningfully through my competencies and dedication to laboratory excellence, while continuing to develop and progress within the Trust.

Question 34:

What is the difference between Band 5 and Band 6?

Background:

Within the NHS, the band system ensures pay and responsibilities are matched fairly to staff experience, competence, and accountability. In pathology, Biomedical Scientists progress from Band 5 (often newly qualified or developing practitioners) to Band 6 (specialist practitioners with greater technical expertise, autonomy, and responsibility). This question is designed to test whether you understand how expectations change between the two bands, both in terms of technical duties and professional responsibilities.

Points to consider:

- What the NHS banding system is
- Overall expectations for Band 5
- Overall expectations for Band 6
- Practical examples across different laboratory departments

Answer:

The NHS banding system is a structured pay and responsibility framework designed to ensure fairness between different roles based on the level of skill, experience, and accountability required. In the pathology laboratory, the progression from Band 5 to Band 6 represents not only an increase in technical competence but also in leadership, autonomy, and contribution to service development.

A Band 5 Biomedical Scientist is usually newly qualified or developing in their career. At this stage, the focus is on building competence across core laboratory functions such as sample reception, routine testing, analyser operation, and basic troubleshooting. Band 5 staff are expected to follow established protocols, validate routine results, and escalate more complex or unusual cases to senior colleagues. **For example, in biochemistry**, a Band 5 might process routine electrolyte and liver function tests, perform analyser maintenance, and validate results within normal or expected ranges, but would escalate unusual endocrine results or troubleshooting beyond first-line checks.

A Band 6 Biomedical Scientist is typically more experienced and competent, often having completed the IBMS Specialist Portfolio or equivalent. This role requires a higher level of autonomy, decision-making, and specialist analytical skills. Band 6 staff are also expected to support the development of Band 5 colleagues through training and mentoring, as well as contributing to audits, quality management, and ongoing service improvement. In haematology, for example, a Band 6 may take responsibility for specialised investigations such as thrombophilia screens, lupus anticoagulant testing, or factor assays, and provide interpretative comments that assist clinicians in managing their patients. They may also lead on troubleshooting analyser issues, perform root cause analysis for QC failures, and liaise directly with clinical teams when urgent or complex results require immediate communication.

In blood transfusion, a Band 5 may competently perform routine blood group, antibody screening, and crossmatch procedures under supervision. However, a Band 6 would take responsibility during major haemorrhage protocols, authorise the issue of complex blood products, investigate antibody problems, and ensure documentation complies with MHRA and ISO15189 standards. They may also train juniors in traceability procedures and manage stock levels proactively.

In microbiology, a Band 5 might focus on routine culture and sensitivity testing, logging samples, and preparing microscopy slides, while escalating unusual isolates. A Band 6, however, would take responsibility for complex identifications such as resistant organisms, validating molecular test results, and supporting outbreak investigations alongside infection control.

In histology, a Band 5 may embed tissues, cut sections, and stain slides, whereas a Band 6 could be expected to perform specialist immunohistochemistry, troubleshoot staining problems, and supervise junior staff in embedding and microtomy.

Overall, the difference between Band 5 and Band 6 is not only technical but also professional. Band 5s focus on developing competence and delivering accurate routine testing, while Band 6s demonstrate specialist expertise, leadership, training responsibilities, and a greater role in quality assurance and audit.

Summary:

A Band 5 Biomedical Scientist is generally at a developing stage, focusing on routine sample analysis, following established protocols, and escalating complex issues to senior staff. In contrast, Band 6 is expected to demonstrate specialist expertise, take greater responsibility for decision-making, lead complex testing, troubleshoot analytical and instrumentation problems, mentor junior colleagues, and contribute actively to audits and quality management. For example, in haematology, Band 5 may validate routine full blood counts, whereas Band 6 would undertake specialised investigations such as thrombophilia testing. Similarly, in blood transfusion, a Band 5 may issue routine crossmatches, while a Band 6 would manage a major haemorrhage call and communicate directly with clinical teams.

The transition reflects not only greater technical competence but also enhanced responsibility for patient safety and service improvement.

Question 35:

What three (3) qualities should a team have for them to achieve the goal?

Background:

As part of a pathology laboratory, teamwork is essential not only among biomedical scientists but also with clinicians, nurses, and other healthcare professionals. Given the diverse cultural and professional backgrounds, teams must build synergy by relying on key qualities that ensure efficiency, accuracy, and patient-centred care. This question is testing your awareness of those vital qualities that enhance collaboration and allow the team to achieve common goals for the benefit of patients.

Points to consider:

- Understanding of the complex and dynamic nature of pathology laboratories and the wider hospital setting.
- Key skills and qualities that enhance teamwork, collaboration, and patient-focused outcomes.
- Practical examples of how these qualities have been demonstrated in practice.

Answer:

While many qualities are important for a team to succeed, I believe the three most vital are effective communication, collaboration and coordination, and mutual trust and respect.

Effective communication ensures that everyone in the team is on the same page, especially in high-pressure situations. For example, in haematology, I was once on a busy evening shift when an analyser broke down. I quickly communicated the issue to colleagues and informed the wards that samples would be processed manually or diverted to another site. Because communication was timely and clear, we avoided confusion, prioritised urgent samples, and maintained patient safety.

Collaboration and coordination allow the workload to be shared effectively so that no single person is overwhelmed. In microbiology, when a blood culture flagged positive.

I worked closely with a colleague to manage the workflow efficiently. For example, while I performed the Gram stain and microscopy, they prepared the sub-cultures. This division of tasks allowed us to work in parallel and deliver preliminary results to clinicians much more quickly, enabling timely treatment decisions. Without this coordination, the process would have taken longer and could have led to avoidable delays.

Mutual trust and respect create a positive work culture where team members value each other's contributions. In transfusion, I once worked with a colleague to resolve a serological ABO discrepancy. We initially had different approaches, but by respecting each other's perspective and working through the process together, we achieved the correct outcome. This not only prevented potential patient harm but also reinforced our teamwork and trust in each other's judgment.

Summary:

In my experience, effective communication, collaboration and coordination, and mutual trust and respect are the three qualities that enable a laboratory team to achieve its goals. These qualities ensure that even under pressure, the team can work together efficiently, maintain laboratory standards, and provide accurate and timely results for the benefit of patient care.

Question 36:

If you have anything to change in your current place of work and how will you change it?

Background:

While the main purpose of the pathology laboratory is to support timely, effective, and accurate patient diagnosis and management, internal challenges can sometimes hinder both service delivery and staff wellbeing. Interviewers want to see if you can critically identify such areas, suggest practical solutions, and balance improvements in efficiency with maintaining quality standards. This does not need to be confined only to technical issues, but can include staffing, training, or workflow organisation.

Points to consider:

- Noticeable challenges that directly or indirectly affect laboratory service.
- Practical examples of problems that have occurred and how they impact patients and staff.
- Constructive recommendations for improvements that would benefit both staff and patient care.

Answer:

In my current workplace, one of the major challenges I have noticed is the high workload coupled with limited staffing, which often leads to increased pressure on the team and affects work-life balance. For example, I have often had to cover weekend shifts almost back-to-back due to staff shortages, and I have seen colleagues become fatigued and demotivated as a result. This impacts team morale and, if not managed carefully, can also increase the risk of errors. Recognising this has reinforced the importance of good communication, fair workload distribution, and supporting one another during high-pressure periods.

Another area I would like to change is the pace and structure of training new staff. In my experience, new biomedical scientists can take a long time to become competent enough to join the shift rota, which leaves the burden on a few trained staff. For instance, I once had to stay beyond my shift to finish pending work because newly appointed colleagues were not yet confident in using the analyser independently. A more structured and accelerated training programme with regular competency assessments would help staff feel supported while also bringing them onto the rota more quickly.

There is also the issue of equipment capacity and reliability. Some of our analysers are older models that frequently give error messages or require repeated troubleshooting. In haematology, I experienced a situation where the analyser flagged errors multiple times within one evening shift, delaying urgent results. Similarly, in biochemistry, delays occur because high-volume analysers cannot keep up with demand at peak times. These equipment issues extend turnaround times and add unnecessary stress. Replacing or upgrading analysers with higher-capacity models would significantly improve workflow and reduce downtime.

My recommendation would be twofold: **first,** to secure funding to employ an adequate number of competent staff, ideally a mix of experienced biomedical scientists and newly qualified staff, so that training and workload can be balanced. **Second,** to invest in more modern analysers with larger higher capacity and better reliability features, which would reduce repetitive breakdowns and streamline the testing process. Together, these improvements would ease staff pressure, enhance morale, and, most importantly, ensure faster and more reliable results for patient care.

Summary:

If I could change something in my current workplace, it would be to address staffing shortages and outdated equipment. By introducing a well-balanced mix of skilled staff and investing in higher-capacity analysers, the laboratory could reduce pressure on individuals, accelerate training, and improve turnaround times. These changes would benefit both staff wellbeing and patient outcomes, ensuring that the laboratory consistently delivers safe, accurate, and timely results.

Question 37:

Where do you see yourself and biomedical scientist (BMS) as a profession in the next 2–5 years?

Background:

It is natural that individuals expect to continue improving in their workplace and professional journey. Biomedical science as a profession has also been evolving, shaped by technological advances, regulatory standards, and the growing recognition of its impact on healthcare. This question is testing whether your ambition lies within the profession or outside, and if you understand the direction the profession is heading in 2–5 years. Your answer should show passion for the profession, highlight your expected growth, and link how your progression will benefit the Trust and patient care.

Points to consider:

- Your passion about the profession
- Your progress within the profession so far
- Your expected development in the coming years
- How that progression benefits the Trust and service delivery
- Observations of the direction of the profession
- If negative trends are identified, provide practical examples of what can be done to address them

Answer:

I have always enjoyed working as a biomedical scientist, and I feel proud to be part of a profession that contributes so significantly to patient care behind the scenes. Over the years, I have progressed steadily within the profession, starting as a trainee and now working confidently as an upper band 5. In the next 1–2 years, I aim to complete my specialist portfolio and progress to band 6, where I will be able to take on more responsibility, including supporting advanced investigations, training new staff, and contributing to laboratory audits and quality improvement projects. Looking further ahead, within 5 years I would like to see myself as a senior biomedical scientist, where I can not only contribute to service delivery but also mentor colleagues, support UKAS inspections, and play a more active role in developing departmental protocols.

From a wider professional perspective, I believe biomedical science will continue to evolve over the next two to five years, with increasing reliance on automation, molecular diagnostics, and digital pathology. These trends are already becoming evident across many laboratory departments

For example**, in biochemistry,** mass spectrometry and high-capacity analysers are increasingly replacing manual or semi-automated methods, improving both accuracy and turnaround times for tests such as toxicology and endocrinology. Biomedical scientists are central to validating these results and troubleshooting instruments when complex faults occur.

In haematology and transfusion, advances in automation mean analysers now detect abnormal cells more accurately, but biomedical scientists remain crucial in interpreting complex cases such as leukaemia flags or antibody identifications. In fact, the growing role of molecular haematology, such as testing for JAK2 and BCR-ABL mutations, is likely to expand the profession's skill set in the coming years.

In microbiology, molecular platforms such as PCR and MALDI-TOF are transforming the speed of organism identification and resistance detection. For instance, rapid tuberculosis testing or same-day MRSA detection is reducing turnaround times dramatically. Biomedical scientists play a key role in verifying these results and ensuring they are communicated promptly to clinical teams.

In histopathology, the growing use of digital pathology and slide scanning is already changing the workflow. In the next few years, biomedical scientists may have more responsibility in digital archiving, slide quality management, and even preliminary image analysis, ensuring that pathologists have the highest quality material to review.

While these innovations are exciting, I also recognise challenges such as increasing workloads and staffing shortages, which can impact service delivery and staff wellbeing. If not addressed, these issues could limit the profession's growth. Personally, I am committed to supporting training and competency development in my workplace so that new staff can integrate into the rota more quickly and contribute effectively. For example, I have been involved in helping trainees with basic analyser maintenance and QC interpretation, which not only builds their confidence but also helps reduce the workload for the wider team.

Summary:

I see myself in the next 2–5 years developing into a more senior role within biomedical science, equipped to train, lead, and support the team, while also contributing to maintaining the Trust's high standards. At the same time, I believe the profession will continue to raise its profile through technological innovation, stronger involvement in clinical pathways, and greater recognition of the vital role biomedical scientists play in patient care.

Question 38:

How will you resolve conflict in your laboratory?

Background:

Conflict is a natural part of any workplace, especially in a pathology laboratory where individuals from different cultural, educational, and professional backgrounds must collaborate in a fast-paced, high-pressure environment. While disagreements can occur, it is important to manage them constructively to ensure they do not affect laboratory performance, staff wellbeing, or, ultimately, patient safety. This question assesses whether you understand how to navigate conflict by prioritising communication, professionalism, and the maintenance of laboratory standards.

Points to consider:

- Understand the dynamic and complex nature of the pathology lab, which attracts people from diverse backgrounds.
- Recognise that conflict often arises from miscommunication or misunderstandings rather than malice.
- Focus on strategies that maintain laboratory quality and patient safety despite differences.
- Provide practical examples of how you have handled or would handle conflict.

Answer:

I believe conflict in the laboratory should always be approached with professionalism and a focus on maintaining service quality. From my experience, most conflicts are the result of miscommunication or differences in expectations, often heightened by the stress of a high workload. When faced with such situations, I make a conscious effort to listen carefully to all parties involved, showing empathy and respect. This often helps to diffuse tension as people feel heard and understood. Once the issue is clear, I focus on finding a solution that supports both teamwork and laboratory standards, because ultimately our common goal is delivering accurate and timely results for patients.

For example, **in haematology,** I once witnessed a disagreement between colleagues regarding the handling of urgent coagulation samples. One member felt another had overlooked a critical sample in favour of routine work. Instead of taking sides, I encouraged both to pause, explained the standard operating procedure for urgent samples, and reassured them that following it would resolve the immediate issue and prevent similar misunderstandings in the future. By shifting the focus back to patient care, the tension quickly eased.

In microbiology, conflict can sometimes arise over workload distribution, especially during busy flu or COVID-19 seasonsI recall a situation where a colleague felt overwhelmed by the number of respiratory samples allocated to them. I stepped in to redistribute tasks more fairly and offered to assist with plate reading. This not only resolved the immediate issue but also fostered a sense of teamwork and collaboration within the laboratory.

In biochemistry, there was a case where a staff member felt that their troubleshooting suggestions for a malfunctioning analyser were not being valued. I helped by facilitating a calm discussion where each person could share their approach. Interestingly, combining both perspectives led us to identify the root of the analyser fault more efficiently. This taught me that encouraging open communication can turn conflict into an opportunity for problem-solving.

In histopathology, differing opinions may occur between biomedical scientists and pathologists regarding the adequacy of specimen processing. I have found that calmly explaining the technical reasoning. For example, tissue fixation times or embedding protocols can reduce misunderstandings and ensure everyone works towards the same goal of producing high-quality diagnostic slides.

Summary:

I handle conflict by listening, clarifying, and redirecting the discussion towards our shared responsibility: delivering safe, accurate, and timely results for patients. Conflict is inevitable in a dynamic laboratory, but when managed constructively, it can strengthen teamwork, improve communication, and enhance service delivery.

Question 39:

You got information about someone being abused, what will you do?

Background:

Pathology laboratories, like all NHS workplaces, are built on values of respect, compassion, and integrity. Abuse in any form whether against patients or staff is unacceptable and against NHS codes of conduct. Abuse may be physical, emotional, verbal, neglect, or even professional misconduct that creates inequalities or unsafe environments.

This question is assessing your understanding of safeguarding, your duty to speak up, and your ability to respond appropriately while prioritising safety, fairness, and patient care.

Points to consider:

- Understanding NHS values and safeguarding responsibilities against abuse, neglect, or any form of discrimination.
- The potential impact of unprofessional behaviour on staff wellbeing, teamwork, and ultimately laboratory quality.
- Knowing and following appropriate escalation channels (line manager, safeguarding lead, freedom to speak up guardian, etc.).
- Practical examples of how you have responded or would respond to such behaviour.

Answer:

Abuse or unprofessional behaviour has no place in the NHS, and it is everyone's responsibility to challenge or report it. My priority would always be to safeguard the individual involved, whether that is a patient, colleague, or another staff member, and to make sure that the correct procedures are followed so the situation is properly investigated.

If I were to get information about someone being abused, my first step would be to remain calm, listen carefully, and not dismiss or minimise the concern. I would then follow the proper reporting channels. If the alleged abuser is a colleague, I would escalate the matter immediately to my line manager or senior staff. If the allegation involved a manager, I would report it directly to another senior leader, the hospital's safeguarding team, or the Freedom to Speak Up Guardian. In situations where there is immediate risk of harm, I would not hesitate to escalate urgently through safeguarding services or even contact emergency services (999) if required.

For example, in one workplace I encountered a situation where a colleague repeatedly used dismissive and belittling language towards a junior member of staff. While it was not physical abuse, it created a hostile environment and was negatively affecting the junior colleague's confidence and performance.

I documented what I observed and raised the matter discreetly with a senior manager. The issue was taken seriously, addressed through HR processes, and eventually led to a healthier working environment for the team.

Another example is in the context of patients' safeguarding. In microbiology, I once received a sample from an elderly patient that came with clinical notes suggesting unexplained recurrent infections and possible neglect. While my role was limited to the laboratory side, I immediately ensured the sample was processed urgently and flagged the notes to my manager, who passed it on to the safeguarding team for follow-up. This demonstrated that abuse or neglect can sometimes be identified indirectly, even from lab data, and must always be acted upon.

Summary:

I understand that abuse in any form cannot be ignored. My role is not to investigate but to report concerns promptly through the appropriate safeguarding channels. By doing so, I contribute to upholding NHS values of compassion and respect, while ensuring the safety and wellbeing of both patients and colleagues.

Question 40:

If one of your calibrators is giving low value, what steps will you take to troubleshoot it?

Background:

Calibrators are reference materials with assigned values used to generate a calibration curve on an analyser. This curve establishes the relationship between instrument signal and analyte concentration, ensuring that patient results are measured accurately and reproducibly. A low calibrator value can compromise the sensitivity and reliability of results, leading to incorrect interpretation of normal, abnormal-low, or abnormal-high ranges. According to ISO15189 and laboratory quality standards, no calibration curve with abnormalities should be accepted without investigation. This question is testing whether you know how to recognise, investigate, and troubleshoot calibration issues to maintain reliability and patient safety.

Points to consider:

- What calibrators are and why they are important in analytical reliability.
- Factors that can affect calibrator values (reagent issues, analyser performance, environmental conditions, handling errors).
- Investigative steps to identify the root cause of low calibrator values.
- Practical troubleshooting examples.

Answer:

If one of my calibrators gave a low value, I would not proceed with patient testing until I had thoroughly investigated and resolved the issue. Accepting a faulty calibration could affect the analyser's sensitivity and lead to unreliable results, which would compromise patient care.

My first step would be to confirm that the calibrator had been prepared, stored, and handled correctly. For example, if it was a reconstituted calibrator, I would check that it had been reconstituted using the correct diluent, mixed thoroughly, and used within the manufacturer's recommended stability period. I would also verify the expiry date and storage conditions, as calibrators are often sensitive to temperature and light.

Next, I would review whether the issue was isolated to one calibrator or affecting the whole calibration curve. If it was only one calibrator level showing low results, it could suggest pipetting errors, improper mixing, or deterioration of that vial. I would repeat the calibration with a fresh vial of the same calibrator to confirm reproducibility.

If the problem persisted, I would then consider analyser-related factors. This might include checking for clots, bubbles, or blockages in the pipetting system, running maintenance (such as probe cleaning or decontamination cycles), and reviewing error logs for instrument malfunctions. For example, **in haematology,** I once encountered a low calibrator for haemoglobin measurement. After reloading fresh calibrator and repeating with the same outcome, I discovered that the photometer lamp was underperforming and required replacement. Once maintenance was performed, the calibration returned within expected values.

I would also review whether reagent lot numbers were correct and consistent with the calibrator lot in use. Sometimes lot-to-lot variations or mismatched reagents can cause calibration drift. For example, **in coagulation,** I have seen a low calibrator caused by expired reagent lots being accidentally left on the analyser. Replacing with in-date reagents and rerunning corrected the curve.

In biochemistry, a low calibrator value could occur in tests such as serum creatinine or electrolytes. For example, I experienced a situation where the lowest calibrator in a creatinine assay gave persistently low readings. Investigation showed that the reagent pack had expired, leading to reduced sensitivity. Once the reagent was replaced with an in-date lot, the calibrator values normalised, and the calibration curve was accepted.

In immunology, I have seen low calibrator results during calibration for hormone assays (e.g., TSH or cortisol). In one instance, the issue was traced back to poor mixing during reconstitution, leaving concentrated material at the bottom of the vial. Proper mixing with gentle inversion resolved the issue, and the calibration curve then fitted within acceptable limits.

Finally, if the problem could not be resolved, I would escalate the issue by logging it in the maintenance system and contacting the manufacturer or engineer for further troubleshooting. In these cases, I would ensure that the analyser is taken out of use until calibration is successful and quality control results are stable.

Summary:

My approach would be systematic: check calibrator preparation and expiry, repeat with a new vial, verify analyser function and maintenance, confirm reagent integrity, and escalate to manufacturer support if needed. This ensures that only a valid calibration is accepted, maintaining ISO15189 standards and guaranteeing reliable patient results.

Question 41:

Example of quality manuals.

Background:

One of the frameworks of quality management system (QMS) in the pathology laboratory is documentation. In addition to the principle that anything not documented is considered not done, documentation serves as a guide to ensure consistency in practice, adherence to standards, and compliance with ISO 15189. Quality manuals define the framework of the Quality Management System and are supported by a range of documents, including Standard Operating Procedures (SOPs), policies, competency records, and audit documentation. This question is assessing your understanding of quality manuals and examples of documentation that support laboratory quality.

Points to consider:

- Quality management system
- Internal documentation
- Examples of documentation that support QMS
- Practical examples of how you have used these in maintaining laboratory quality

Answer:

Quality manuals are essential in pathology laboratories because they provide a structured framework for implementing, monitoring, and maintaining quality in line with ISO15189 and UKAS standards. A quality manual is a top-level document that describes the laboratory's quality policies, processes, and objectives, setting out how quality is embedded into every aspect of laboratory practice.

Examples of documents that fall under the scope of quality manuals include:

- **Standard Operating Procedures (SOPs):** These describe in detail how each test or process should be performed, ensuring consistency across all staff members. For example, in haematology, I have used the SOP for full blood count analysis to ensure I follow the same process for sample loading, running QC, and validating results as every other member of staff.

- **Quality Control (QC) and Quality Assurance (QA) records:** These document daily checks on analysers, control results, and corrective actions when QC falls outside acceptable ranges. For instance, in biochemistry, I regularly record QC performance in accordance with Westgard rules, documenting investigations when controls fail.

- **Competency and training records:** These ensure staff have been trained and deemed competent for specific procedures. In my current role, I ensure my competency records are up to date and that I sign training logs after completing refresher training, which is crucial during UKAS audits.

- **Audit reports:** Internal audit records are part of the quality manual framework and ensure ongoing compliance with ISO15189. For example, during a recent internal audit in microbiology, I helped check documentation for antimicrobial susceptibility testing, making sure that maintenance and QC records were available and up to date.

- **Incident and non-conformance records:** These are used to record deviations from standard procedures. In histology, for example, if a specimen was mislabelled, an incident form would be raised and corrective action documented to prevent recurrence.

By using these documents in practice, I have seen how the quality manual system ensures traceability, accountability, and consistency. For example, when preparing for an external UKAS inspection, I supported the team by verifying that all SOPs were current, properly signed, and version-controlled, ensuring full compliance with the Quality Management System requirements.

Summary:

Quality manuals provide the foundation of the QMS by detailing policies, objectives, and responsibilities while being supported by SOPs, QC/QA records, training logs, audit reports, and incident records. I have actively used these documents in haematology, microbiology, biochemistry, and histology to ensure quality and compliance, and to prepare for both internal and external audits. This demonstrates how proper documentation directly supports patient safety and laboratory efficiency.

Question 42:

Explain how you can work on a 24/7 shift roster.

Background:

Most pathology laboratories operate 24 hours a day, 7 days a week, and 365 days a year. This ensures that urgent diagnostic services are always available to support patient care, whether in A&E, ITU, maternity, or wards. As a result, biomedical scientists are expected to participate in a shift system, including nights, weekends, and bank holidays. Out-of-hours shifts often mean working as a lone worker or with limited staff, so it is vital to maintain standards, manage workload effectively, and know when and how to escalate issues. This question tests your awareness of the requirements of a 24/7 rota, your understanding of lone working, and your ability to ensure quality under such conditions.

Points to consider:

- Pathology laboratory out-of-hours shift or rota
- Challenges and benefits of out-of-hours lone working
- Quality management system

Answer:

I understand that most pathology laboratories run a 24/7 shift system, and I am fully prepared to work within such a rota. Out-of-hours cover is essential, as urgent and emergency requests cannot be delayed. These include blood transfusion for major haemorrhage, urgent biochemistry tests for suspected sepsis, and emergency CSF analysis for possible meningitis.

One of the key challenges of working out of hours is being a lone worker or part of a very small team. This means I may have to handle urgent requests, troubleshoot analysers, communicate with clinical staff, and maintain documentation all at once. For example, during a night shift **in haematology,** I once had to manage a major haemorrhage call while simultaneously troubleshooting an analyser that failed QC. I followed the SOPs, performed manual crossmatching, and liaised directly with the clinical team to ensure that safe blood was issued without delay.

Similarly, **in biochemistry,** I have worked night shifts where analyser downtime required me to switch to backup equipment and liaise with the on-call engineer. In these situations, maintaining a calm and methodical approach is vital, documenting each step and prioritising urgent samples such as those for ITU or A&E.

In microbiology, out-of-hours shifts often involve urgent Gram stains or MRSA screening. On one occasion, a maternity ward requested urgent Group B Streptococcus screening. Although full culture would take longer, I followed the SOP to provide an initial report based on rapid testing, ensuring the clinician had timely information for patient management.

Working in this way requires excellent time management, prioritisation, and communication. To maintain quality, I rely heavily on SOPs, document all actions taken, and escalate to the on-call senior or consultant when needed. At the same time, lone working has also given me the opportunity to build confidence in independent decision-making and strengthen my critical thinking skills.

Summary:

I can confidently work on a 24/7 rota, understanding both the challenges and the importance of out-of-hours service. By relying on SOPs, effective communication, prioritisation, and escalation when required, I can maintain high-quality results and patient safety. My experience across haematology, biochemistry, and microbiology demonstrates that I am capable of handling lone-working situations while ensuring compliance with ISO15189 and supporting urgent patient care.

Question 43:

Your band 6 has refused to put in a word for you for promotion, how will you go about it?

Background:

It is normal for staff to expect recognition and progression in their career, and sometimes this may involve support from a senior colleague or manager. However, the decision to promote often goes beyond one individual's recommendation and depends on competence, experience, and Trust processes. This question tests your ability to manage disappointment calmly, focus on professionalism, and pursue constructive alternatives while maintaining the quality of your work.

Points to note:

- Regulate emotions and feelings
- Explore other legal and professional options
- Focus on improving competence

Answer:

If I found myself in a situation where my band 6 declined to put in a word for my promotion, I would remain calm and professional. While it is natural to feel disappointed, I believe it is important not to allow emotions to negatively affect the quality of my work or my relationship with colleagues.

My first step would be to politely request feedback from my band 6 to understand their reasons. For example, they may feel I need to strengthen certain competencies, such as leadership or advanced troubleshooting. Having this feedback would give me the opportunity to work on those areas and demonstrate improvement over time.

If I still felt that I was ready for promotion, I would explore other legitimate options. For example, I could raise the matter with my line manager or another senior colleague, ensuring I communicate in a respectful and professional manner. I would also ensure that such discussions are documented. For instance, by following up with an email after a conversation to keep a clear record of the steps I have taken.

At the same time, I would remain committed to maintaining high standards in my current role. For example, I have supported junior colleagues in learning analyser maintenance and interpreting quality control results. By recording these contributions, I can demonstrate clear evidence of my readiness to take on greater responsibility.

Ultimately, my goal would be to remain committed to patient care and laboratory quality while working on any identified gaps in my competency. I believe that demonstrating consistent professionalism, competence, and dedication to Trust values will strengthen my case for promotion, regardless of whether one particular colleague is supportive.

Summary:

If my band 6 refused to support my promotion, I would stay calm, seek constructive feedback, and explore alternative professional channels such as discussing with another senior or manager. Meanwhile, I would continue building my competence and documenting contributions to strengthen my case. This ensures that I remain professional, focused on service quality, and proactive in my career progression.

Question 44:

How will you run a haemolysed sample and what additional test can be done?

Background:

Haemolysis can occur due to pre-analytical errors (e.g., incorrect phlebotomy technique, inappropriate centrifugation, or delayed sample separation) or due to underlying physiological conditions such as autoimmune haemolytic anaemia. While some laboratories may accept mildly haemolysed samples for limited testing, in most cases haemolysis interferes with results and renders them unreliable. This question tests whether you understand how to apply laboratory SOPs, make appropriate scientific decisions, and consider follow-up testing to investigate possible pathological haemolysis.

Points to consider:

- Laboratory SOP
- Scientific decision-making
- Required action
- Practical examples

Answer:

If I receive a haemolysed sample, my first step would be to assess the degree of haemolysis and follow the laboratory SOP. In most cases, haemolysed samples are rejected because the destruction of red blood cells releases intracellular components such as potassium, LDH, and AST into the serum or plasma, leading to falsely elevated results. Similarly, haemolysis can cause falsely low haptoglobin due to consumption. This poses a serious risk to patient safety, as clinical decisions may be made on inaccurate results.

Therefore, my approach would be to reject the haemolysed sample and request a repeat from the clinical team, explaining clearly why the sample is unsuitable. At the same time, if the haemolysis is suspected to be physiological rather than artefactual, I would discuss with the requesting clinician and consider further investigations to establish the underlying cause.

For example:

In **Biochemistry**, haemolysis can interfere with tests such as potassium, bilirubin, ALT, LDH, and troponin. If physiological haemolysis is suspected, additional tests including haptoglobin, bilirubin (especially the unconjugated fraction), and LDH can help support the assessment.

In **Haematology**, if immune-mediated haemolysis is a concern, a Direct Antiglobulin Test (DAT/Coombs test) may be appropriate to investigate autoimmune causes. A reticulocyte count and blood film examination can provide further supporting evidence.

In **Blood Transfusion**, a haemolysed sample may be unsuitable for group and screen or crossmatch, as haemolysis can mask antibody detection or obscure signs of a haemolytic transfusion reaction. A repeat sample would therefore be required.

In **Microbiology**, although haemolysis itself is less directly relevant, a compromised or contaminated blood sample can affect culture reliability. In such cases, a repeat sample would also be requested.

A practical example from my experience: I once received a potassium result >10 mmol/L on a grossly haemolysed sample. Instead of validating, I immediately rejected the sample, phoned the ward, and explained that the haemolysis likely accounted for the abnormal value. A repeat sample was collected and analysed, and the potassium came back within the normal range, preventing unnecessary escalation to critical care.

Summary:

Haemolysed samples are generally rejected under SOP guidelines to prevent false results and potential patient mismanagement. However, if physiological haemolysis is suspected, further tests such as LDH, bilirubin, haptoglobin, reticulocyte count, and DAT may be performed to investigate the cause. By balancing adherence to SOPs with good scientific reasoning and clear communication with clinicians, I ensure both patient safety and diagnostic accuracy.

Question 45:

How can you encourage a team to improve?

Background:

Pathology laboratories rely heavily on teamwork, as each stage of the diagnostic pathway from sample reception, analysis, validation, and reporting is interlinked. A breakdown in teamwork can slow turnaround times, reduce accuracy, or negatively affect staff morale. Factors such as workload pressures, interpersonal differences, or communication barriers can weaken team spirit. This question assesses how you would actively contribute to sustaining and improving team effectiveness, always with patient safety and laboratory quality at the centre.

Points to consider:

- Importance of laboratory teamwork
- Factors that could affect the team
- How you would contribute to team focus on quality
- Practical examples

Answer:

I believe that a strong, motivated team is essential for delivering accurate, timely, and reliable results that directly support patient care. When encouraging a team to improve, my first step is to highlight our shared goal: upholding high laboratory standards for the benefit of patients. Connecting everyday tasks to real patient outcomes reinforces our sense of purpose and helps the team stay focused and engaged.

I would also address factors that can weaken team spirit, such as uneven workload distribution or lack of communication. For example, ensuring that rotas are fairly balanced to support work-life balance can significantly improve morale. I would encourage open communication during handovers, so colleagues feel supported, and problems are resolved early. Small gestures, like acknowledging good work, can also go a long way in encouraging colleagues.

Example:

In Haematology: I once worked with a team under pressure during staff shortages. To keep morale up, I encouraged team members to rotate between high-pressure tasks such as blood film reporting and more routine automated work, so no one felt overwhelmed. This improved efficiency and prevented errors due to fatigue.

In Biochemistry: During a UKAS inspection preparation, I motivated colleagues by suggesting we break tasks into manageable sections and share responsibility. By focusing on strengths, while some are updating SOPs, others were preparing evidence for traceability. The coordination helped us to complete the preparation ahead of time, which boosted confidence across the team.

In Blood Transfusion: When tensions rose during an urgent crossmatch for a trauma case, I encouraged calm coordination by reminding the team of our training, assigning clear roles, and providing reassurance. This kept us focused and allowed us to deliver life-saving blood products quickly and safely.

Summary:

I would encourage a team to improve by maintaining focus on patient-centred laboratory quality, addressing issues that affect morale, and fostering open communication and mutual support. By promoting fairness in rotas, recognising individual contributions, and encouraging collaboration, I can help the team stay motivated, efficient, and aligned with the Trust's values.

Question 46:

What are your weaknesses and how does your strength complement your weaknesses?

Background:

Teamwork is the hallmark of pathology laboratories, where weaknesses in one area can often be balanced by the strengths of other colleagues, and vice versa. This question is testing whether you are aware of your own areas for improvement, how you use your strengths to balance them, and how you contribute to the team while also being open to support.

Point to consider:

- Understanding of the importance of teamwork
- Awareness of how you can contribute to the team
- Awareness of areas where you may rely on the team
- Practical examples of how you use your strengths to compensate for your weaknesses

Answer:

One weakness I have recognised in myself is that I sometimes try to handle too much on my own before asking for help. This comes from a desire to remain dependable and ensure high standards, but I have realised that it is not always the most efficient or collaborative approach, especially in a busy pathology laboratory where teamwork is vital. To overcome this, I actively use my strength in communication and my willingness to support others. I have learned to let colleagues know when I may require assistance and to involve the team earlier, rather than taking everything on myself.

For example, during a particularly busy out-of-hours shift in biochemistry, several urgent requests arrived at the same time as routine samples, and I initially tried to handle everything on my own. When I realised this was affecting turnaround times, I communicated clearly with my colleagues, delegated appropriate tasks, and focused on the urgent work. This collaborative approach ensured that patient care was not delayed and reinforced to me that teamwork is far more effective than working in isolation.

In haematology, when troubleshooting a complex analyser error that was slowing down urgent samples, I used my strength in problem-solving but also called on the experience of a senior colleague to double-check my conclusions. My willingness to seek help ensured that I avoided unnecessary delays and maintained quality standards.

In microbiology, I have the opposite experience: colleagues often rely on me to support with documentation and communication with clinicians because of my strength in clarity and organisation. This means that while I may lean on the team for technical advice in some situations, I balance it by contributing my own strengths in areas where I excel.

Overall, I see my weaknesses as opportunities for growth, and I use my strengths such as communication, teamwork, and problem-solving to ensure that they do not impact patient care or laboratory standards.

Summary:

One of my weaknesses is that I sometimes take on too much work before asking for help. I have been addressing this by using my strong communication skills to share updates, seek support earlier, and ensure tasks are completed on time. My strengths in organisation, multitasking, and teamwork complement this, as they enable me to support colleagues, troubleshoot efficiently, and maintain high standards across departments. This balance allows me to turn a potential weakness into an opportunity for growth while keeping patient safety and quality at the centre of my practice.

Question 47:

How do you ensure a person is working on the machine like every other person?

Background:

According to ISO15189 recommendations, staff are only permitted to perform tasks within their areas of demonstrated competence. This requires structured training, competency assessments, and formal sign-off before independent use of laboratory equipment. Even after competency is established, continued assurance is maintained through internal audits, observations, and refresher training. Reporting and addressing non-conformance are also key to ensuring patient safety and maintaining laboratory standards. This question is testing your understanding of how training, competency, audits, and quality assurance measures ensure that all staff operate analysers to the same high standard.

Points to consider:

- ISO15189 recommendations on competency
- Training and competency sign-off
- Ongoing examination and audit
- Reporting non-conformance
- Practical examples

Answer:

Ensuring that every staff member works consistently on an analyser requires structured training, competency assessments, and ongoing quality monitoring, all in line with ISO15189. This means that no one is allowed to operate equipment independently until they have completed training, been assessed, and signed off as competent. Beyond initial sign-off, audits and periodic re-assessments are conducted to confirm continued adherence to SOPs and maintain uniformity in practice. Where non-conformance is identified, it must be documented, reported, and followed up with retraining.

In haematology, for example, when a new staff member is trained on the Sysmex analyser, they must demonstrate competence in daily QC, sample processing, error troubleshooting, and maintenance documentation. Only once they complete their competency sign-off can they work independently. During one internal audit, incomplete analyser maintenance logs were discovered. This was reported, retraining was organised for the staff involved, and the issue was corrected helping ensure all staff maintained the same standard of practice.

In biochemistry, on the Roche Cobas analyser, training covers calibration, QC interpretation, and reagent management. I once observed a situation where a colleague was handling QC incorrectly, which was flagged during a UKAS visit. The non-conformance report led to refresher training, ensuring the analyser results remained accurate and reproducible.

In microbiology, training on equipment such as MALDI-TOF includes both sample preparation and interpretation of results.

Competency must be renewed periodically. In one case, a staff member's competency reviews highlighted deviation from SOPs in sample preparation. The issue was addressed through retraining, preventing potential errors and ensuring quality was consistent across the team.

These examples demonstrate how training, auditing, and retraining ensure that all staff members, regardless of experience, work to the same standard on laboratory equipment.

Summary:

I ensure that every staff member works on the analyser in the same way through structured training, competency sign-off, and continued audits. These measures are in line with ISO15189 and guarantee that no one works beyond their level of competence. When issues are identified, such as incomplete logs or deviation from SOPs, I make sure they are reported and followed up with retraining. This approach not only maintains consistency across the team but also safeguards patient safety, upholds laboratory standards, and ensures that all analysers deliver accurate and reproducible results.

Question 48:

How will you balance competency training and your commitment to service?

Background:

One of the challenges facing NHS pathology laboratories is balancing training with other required laboratory tasks. Short staffing, emergencies, or equipment downtime can all disrupt planned training sessions. This question tests your ability to plan, prioritise, and ensure both service delivery and staff development continue without compromising laboratory standards.

Points to consider:

- Acknowledge factors that impact training and other laboratory tasks
- Demonstrate the need for effective structured planning and prioritisation
- Provide practical examples

Answer:

Balancing competency training and service delivery requires careful planning and flexibility. In a busy and dynamic pathology laboratory, unforeseen events such as staff absences, equipment failures, or urgent sample processing can disrupt planned activities. For example, if several staff members call in sick, I may need to cover bench work to ensure patient samples are processed without delay.

To manage this, I maintain a training calendar and allocate protected time for competency development. I prioritise training sessions during quieter periods, such as afternoon shifts or days with fewer urgent samples, while ensuring all core laboratory tasks are completed efficiently. If emergencies arise during a training session, I can temporarily pause the session, handle urgent work, and then resume training once the situation is under control.

For instance, while supervising a newly qualified staff member in biochemistry, an urgent request for a critical electrolyte panel came through. I quickly delegated routine tasks to other team members and personally processed the urgent sample, then returned to guide the trainee through their competency exercises. This approach ensures both service continuity and staff development are maintained without compromising patient safety or laboratory quality.

Summary:

Balancing training with service requires structured planning, prioritisation, and flexibility. I maintain a clear training calendar while ensuring core laboratory tasks are completed to standard. In the event of unforeseen circumstances, I can

adjust priorities, delegate tasks, and resume training once the situation stabilises. This approach allows competency development to continue alongside high-quality service delivery, maintaining patient safety and upholding ISO15189 laboratory standards.

Question 49:

Have you been involved in an audit? What role did you play?

Background:

Audit is an essential component of a Quality Management System (QMS) in pathology laboratories, consistent with ISO15189 requirements. Both internal and external audits are conducted to ensure laboratory processes adhere to documented standards and that quality assurance (QA) is maintained. External audits, such as UKAS assessments, evaluate overall laboratory compliance and competence. This question tests your understanding of audits, their purpose, and your practical involvement in them.

Points to consider:

- What an audit is
- Audit and quality assurance
- Role in UKAS assessment or other audits
- Practical examples of audit participation

Answer:

An audit is a systematic evaluation of laboratory processes to determine whether they conform to established standards and documented procedures. It identifies areas of compliance, non-conformance, and opportunities for improvement, ensuring that the laboratory consistently delivers accurate, reliable, and reproducible results. Internal audits can take various forms, such as vertical, horizontal, witness/examination, or clinical audits, while external audits, like UKAS assessments, review the laboratory's overall compliance with ISO15189 standards.

I have been actively involved in several audits across departments. For example, during an internal examination audit in biochemistry, I demonstrated my competency in results validation by explaining how I verified patient results using quality control data and how I recorded and escalated any discrepancies. In haematology, I contributed to an internal audit focused on analyser maintenance and QC reporting, ensuring that all daily, weekly, and monthly maintenance records were accurate, complete, and up to date.

Additionally, I have contributed to UKAS external assessments. In one instance, I guided the auditor through the laboratory, explaining the pre-analytical phase, such as sample reception and logging, and the analytical phase, such as calibrations, controls, and troubleshooting of analysers. I also provided evidence of staff competency records and QC performance, highlighting adherence to SOPs. These experiences allowed me to support the audit process while ensuring the laboratory demonstrated full compliance with regulatory standards.

Summary:

Audits, both internal and external, are crucial for ensuring laboratory quality and compliance with ISO15189. My involvement has included demonstrating competency in results validation, guiding auditors through laboratory processes, and providing evidence of compliance in multiple departments such as biochemistry and haematology. These experiences have reinforced my understanding of the importance of documentation, QC, and continuous quality improvement in maintaining high laboratory standards.

Question 50:

If your colleague's sample was sent in from A & E, what would you do?

Background:

This situation can arise when a member of staff is unwell and admitted through A & E. While it may be tempting to give a colleague's sample special attention, NHS guidelines emphasise equality, inclusiveness, and fairness. This question tests whether you understand that prioritisation should be based on clinical urgency, not personal connections.

Points to consider:

- NHS guidelines and values on equality and inclusiveness
- Adhering to NHS guidelines and values
- Prioritise urgent samples without partiality
- Give practical examples

Answer:

I would prioritise the colleague's sample based on clinical urgency, in the same way as any other urgent sample from A & E, ITU, or the delivery suite. For example, **in biochemistry,** if the colleague's sample is for potassium and renal function tests, I would first process any critically ill patient's sample showing potential life-threatening abnormalities, ensuring results are available in time for urgent clinical decisions.

In haematology, if the colleague's sample is for a full blood count and the ward has a patient with suspected sepsis, I would prioritise the septic patient's sample first, as the clinical outcome could be immediately affected. The colleague's sample would still be processed urgently, but not ahead of another patient in a critical condition.

In microbiology, if the colleague's sample is a blood culture, I would check if any other patient samples were flagged as urgent or suspected of bloodstream infection. I would then process all urgent cultures in the correct order based on clinical need rather than personal familiarity.

By doing this, I ensure adherence to NHS values of equality and inclusiveness, while maintaining fairness and professionalism. It also ensures that urgent patient care is not compromised by personal bias, and all patients are treated equitably.

Summary:

Handling a colleague's sample is treated in exactly the same way as any other urgent request. Clinical urgency, not personal relationships, determines the order of processing. Whether in biochemistry, haematology, or microbiology, I remain focused on maintaining fairness, following NHS guidelines, and ensuring that patient care and laboratory standards are always upheld.

Question 51:

When a colleague hands over to you and you found out that a wrong result was sent out by the colleague, what will you do?

Background:

Pathology laboratories run on a 24/7 basis, making handovers between shifts a critical part of ensuring patient safety and continuity of service. Mistakes can happen, such as an incorrect result being authorised and sent out. While errors are inevitable in any human system, how they are handled is vital. According to ISO15189 and NHS values, any non-conformance must be reported, corrected, and investigated. This not only safeguards patients but also provides learning opportunities for the team and prevents recurrence. This question is testing your understanding on the need to report any non-conformance and whether you are aware why that is important.

Points to consider:

- Importance of thorough handovers in a 24/7 service.

- Identification and correction of non-conformance.
- Reporting via incident forms and escalation.
- Using the error as a learning tool (training, retraining, SOP review).
- Practical examples.

Answer:

Handover is one of the most critical points in laboratory workflow, and part of my role is to carefully review the information given to me to ensure there are no gaps or errors. If I discover that a wrong result has been released, I will first confirm the error by reviewing the analyser data, QC performance, and sample integrity. If the mistake is verified, I would take immediate steps to correct the result on the laboratory system (LIMS) and ensure the amended report is released. At the same time, I would notify the relevant clinician promptly, as delays in correcting errors could negatively impact patient care.

After correction, I would complete an incident form in line with the Trust's incident reporting system (e.g., Datix). This ensures the non-conformance is formally recorded and investigated. Root cause analysis may show whether the error was due to analyser malfunction, misinterpretation, inadequate handover, or even short staffing. The outcome would then guide whether retraining, updating SOPs, or strengthening the handover process is needed.

For example, **in biochemistry,** if a potassium result was incorrectly validated as normal when in fact the patient was hyperkalaemic, this could delay urgent treatment. Correcting the result immediately and contacting the ward would be vital. **In haematology,** if a full blood count showed severe anaemia but was released as normal due to oversight, I would correct the error, alert the clinical team, and document it as an incident. Similarly, **in microbiology**, if a wrong antibiotic sensitivity was reported, it could have major clinical implications. So, I would immediately notify the ward, correct the report, and escalate to my senior.

By approaching the issue in a professional, structured way, I not only protect the patient but also maintain transparency, accountability, and adherence to ISO15189 requirements.

Summary:

If I discovered that a wrong result had been released during handover, I would first verify the error, then correct it immediately and ensure the amended report reached the clinical team without delay. I would also raise an incident report, as transparency and accountability are key to maintaining quality. For example, if a critical potassium in biochemistry or a major haemorrhage sample in haematology was misreported, I would act quickly to correct it and escalate to my manager. I see errors as opportunities for improvement, so I would contribute to the root cause analysis, ensuring lessons are learned and processes such as handovers and SOPs are strengthened to prevent recurrence.

Question 52:

When the IT system fails which affect phones and you need to release results, what would you do?

Background:

Laboratory services rely heavily on IT systems across all phases of testing: the pre-analytical stage, which includes sample collection and booking; the analytical stage, which involves testing and validation; and the post-analytical stage, where results are reported and communicated. IT downtime can significantly disrupt workflow and create risks to patient safety if urgent results are delayed. Therefore, it is essential that laboratory staff follow the downtime SOP, use alternative communication channels, and ensure clear documentation of all actions. This question is testing your understanding on what to do to continue to ensure patients' safety and maintain standards during IT failure.

Points to consider:

- Investigate IT system by troubleshooting.
- Confirm the IT failure by contacting the IT department.
- Use alternative means of hospital communication in such an event.
- Follow SOP to deal with IT downtime.
- Ensure proper documentation of your actions.
- Give practical examples where applicable.

Answer:

IT downtime can be particularly challenging in the laboratory because urgent and critical results often need to be communicated promptly to support patient management. My first step would be to confirm that the issue is a genuine IT failure, which I would do by checking the system locally and contacting the IT department for clarification. While waiting for IT to resolve the problem, I would immediately switch to the downtime SOP, which provides step-by-step guidance on maintaining service delivery when IT systems are unavailable.

For urgent results, such as those requested by A&E, ITU, or the delivery suite, I would print the analyser output and deliver or phone through the results using any available alternative lines. If hospital phones were also down, I would escalate immediately to a manager or senior staff so that backup communication methods could be activated, such as hospital radios, pagers, internal runners, or the secure emergency mobile phones used by some departments. If direct communication with the clinical team were still temporarily impossible despite escalation, I would document the urgency, secure the printed result, and hand-deliver it to the appropriate ward or department as quickly as possible.

For example, **in haematology,** if a critical INR result is generated during downtime, I would print the analyser report and hand-deliver it to A&E or ITU. **In biochemistry**, if potassium levels are dangerously high, I would follow the same approach and escalate directly to the treating ward. **In blood transfusion**, downtime is especially sensitive, as safe issue of blood is paramount. I would follow the manual issue SOP, cross-check records, and deliver units physically to the clinical team while documenting every step to ensure traceability.

In addition, I would ensure all results generated during downtime are properly logged and later uploaded into the LIMS once the IT system is restored, ensuring there are no gaps in the patient's electronic record.

Summary:

If faced with IT downtime that also affects phone systems, I would immediately follow the downtime SOP, confirm the issue with IT, and switch to alternative communication methods to ensure urgent results are delivered safely and on time. For critical tests in haematology, biochemistry, and blood transfusion, I would hand-deliver results or escalate via emergency contacts to prevent any risk to patient care. All actions would be clearly documented, and results would be entered retrospectively once the system is restored. This approach maintains patient safety, supports compliance with ISO 15189, and demonstrates resilience in managing service disruptions.

Question 53:

Sample was sent to the lab not properly labelled and the doctor insists you should process it. What will you do and what action will you take?

Background:

Sometimes samples arrive in the laboratory without proper labelling, often due to oversight at the collection stage. This can be frustrating for clinicians who may try to persuade laboratory staff to process the sample regardless, especially in urgent cases. However, accepting such a sample is against NHS guidelines, quality assurance policies, and ISO15189 recommendations, as it poses significant risk to patient safety and can lead to misidentification, incorrect results, and inappropriate patient management. The only exception to this strict policy is with certain critical samples, such as CSF, where rejecting may mean the loss of an irreplaceable specimen - in such cases, additional safeguards, documentation, and accountability are required. This question is testing your understanding of why unlabelled or mislabelled samples must be rejected, when exceptions apply, and how to use communication skills to politely but firmly explain the policy while maintaining professionalism.

Points to consider:

- Understanding of the NHS labelling policy.
- Importance of strict adherence to ISO15189 and Trust guidelines.
- Quality assurance and patient safety.
- Exception for precious samples like CSF.
- Communication and diplomacy when addressing clinicians.
- Practical examples where applicable.

Answer:

If I receive an unlabelled or mislabelled sample, I will not process it, as doing so would compromise patient safety and go against ISO15189 standards, NHS policy, and our laboratory's SOP. While I may not be in a position to dispute the clinician's claim about where the sample came from, it is my responsibility to ensure that results released are safe, traceable, and accurate.

In such a situation, I would use clear and polite communication to explain to the doctor that the laboratory cannot accept unlabelled or mislabelled samples because of the risk of error. I would reassure them that I fully understand the urgency and importance of the patient's care, and I would encourage them to recollect and correctly label the sample. I would also reassure them that once the properly labelled sample is received, it will be prioritised and processed quickly.

For example, **in biochemistry,** processing an unlabelled potassium sample could lead to inappropriate treatment of hyperkalaemia in the wrong patient. **In haematology,** an unlabelled FBC could result in misdiagnosis of sepsis or anaemia. **In blood transfusion**, an unlabelled crossmatch sample poses one of the highest risks, as issuing blood against the wrong patient could be fatal. Therefore, in most cases, the only safe course of action is to reject and request recollection.

The exception is CSF samples, which are often difficult or impossible to recollect. In this situation, I would contact the requesting clinician immediately, ask them to come to the laboratory, and label the sample in my presence. I would record their full details, including name, signature, and bleep number, and ensure this information is documented in both the patient record and the laboratory system. This approach maintains accountability and full traceability while safeguarding patient safety.

Short scenario (polite communication example):

Doctor: "I know this CSF belongs to my patient - can't you just process it for me?"

Me: "I completely understand your concern, doctor, but our policy and ISO15189 guidelines mean we cannot process unlabelled samples. This protects patient safety and prevents the risk of results being attached to the wrong patient. If this were, for example, a blood sample, I would need to ask you to recollect and resubmit it. However, because this is a CSF and recollection is not straightforward, I can ask you to come to the lab, label the sample in my presence, and sign the documentation so it can be safely processed. That way, we ensure both urgency and patient safety are maintained."

Summary:

If a sample is not properly labelled, I will not process it, as this goes against NHS policy, ISO15189, and laboratory SOPs. I would politely but firmly explain this to the clinician and request a recollected and correctly labelled sample, reassuring them that it will be processed urgently once received. The only exception would be for irreplaceable

samples such as CSF, where I would ask the doctor to attend the lab, label the sample in my presence, and provide their details, ensuring full documentation and accountability. This maintains both patient safety and professional standards while using clear communication to manage a potentially difficult discussion.

Question 54:

What are the benefits of participating in a quality assurance scheme and how should the samples be processed?

Background:

Quality assurance (QA) is a system designed to prevent errors in the laboratory and ensure consistent adherence to required standards. QA schemes are structured programs, which are either internal or external, such as the National External Quality Assessment Service (NEQAS) that help laboratories maintain accuracy, reliability, and compliance with ISO15189. Samples provided through QA schemes must be processed in exactly the same way as patient samples to ensure that the laboratory's procedures are valid and reproducible. This question is testing your understanding of QA programs, the role they play in patient safety, and the importance of treating QA samples with the same method as clinical specimens.

Points to consider:

- What QA and QA schemes are.
- Role of QA in patient safety and standardisation.
- Ensuring QA samples are processed using the same method as patient samples.
- Practical examples where applicable

Answer:

Participating in a QA scheme is essential to ensure that the laboratory maintains high standards and consistently delivers accurate results in line with ISO15189 and SOPs. QA schemes provide an independent benchmark, helping to identify errors, assess staff competency, and confirm that analytical processes are performing correctly. This contributes directly to patient safety, as results generated by the laboratory can be trusted for clinical decision-making.

Samples from external QA programs such as NEQAS should be treated exactly like patient samples. They should be received, logged, processed, analysed, and reported according to the same protocols and quality control measures applied to patient specimens. For example, **in biochemistry,** a NEQAS serum sample for glucose or electrolytes would be processed on the same analyser, following the same QC checks, calibrations, and method verification steps as actual patient samples. **In haematology,** a NEQAS FBC sample would be run on the same analyser, with the same gating and flagging procedures applied. **In microbiology,** an external QA culture or molecular sample should be streaked, incubated, and reported in the same way as routine patient samples to ensure consistency.

From my experience, I was once responsible for processing a NEQAS biochemistry sample during a week where the laboratory was very busy. I ensured the sample was logged correctly, ran it on the analyser using the same pre-analytical and analytical protocols as patient samples, and performed all QC checks before validating the result. I then compared the results to the expected NEQAS ranges and documented the process carefully. This approach ensured compliance with the SOPs and ISO15189 requirements, while also demonstrating to my senior that I could maintain high standards even under pressure.

Internal QA schemes are also valuable. For instance, some laboratories implement cross-site sample testing where a sample is sent to another lab for validation or parallel testing. Daily, weekly, and monthly QC checks also serve as part of the internal QA framework, monitoring analyser performance, reagent integrity, and staff competency. These practices help detect trends that may indicate potential errors before they impact patient results.

Summary:

Participating in a quality assurance scheme ensures that the laboratory maintains accuracy, reliability, and compliance with ISO15189 standards. QA programs, both internal and external, help protect patient safety by identifying errors and confirming that processes and staff performance meet required standards. QA samples must be processed exactly like patient specimens, whether in biochemistry, haematology, or microbiology. From my experience handling NEQAS samples, I consistently ensured correct logging, processing, QC checks, and documentation, which supports ongoing quality improvement and reassures clinicians and patients that laboratory results are accurate.

Question 55:

How do you cope as a lone worker in a high-pressured environment?

Background:

Most pathology laboratories operate 24/7, meaning that staff are sometimes required to cover out-of-hours shifts. During these shifts, the number of staff is limited, and often a biomedical scientist may be the only person present in the laboratory, acting as a lone worker. This responsibility can be challenging, particularly when workload increases, urgent samples arrive, or unexpected issues arise. The question tests your ability to plan, prioritise, multitask, communicate, and maintain attention to detail, all while ensuring that laboratory standards and patient safety are not compromised.

Points to consider:

- Understanding the pressure and responsibilities of lone working.
- Maintaining consistent standards regardless of workload or pressure.
- Practical strategies and examples.

- Personal and professional growth associated with lone working.

Answer:

Working alone in a laboratory can be challenging, especially when workload is high or unexpected events occur. The key is to remain calm, organised, and systematic in approaching the tasks at hand. I start by planning and prioritising my workload based on urgency, clinical impact, and deadlines. For example, urgent samples from A&E, ITU, or maternity wards are processed first, ensuring patient care is supported. Routine samples are scheduled around these priorities without compromising quality.

I rely on strong multitasking skills and attention to detail to ensure that every stage of the process, from sample reception and processing to analysis and result validation, is carried out accurately. In biochemistry, for example, I may be running a critical electrolyte panel while performing QC checks and logging incoming samples. In haematology, I might be manually reviewing flagged FBC results while monitoring analyser performance and confirming that daily controls remain within range. In microbiology, I may be managing culture inoculations and checking identification results while ensuring that urgent CSF or blood cultures are prioritised and processed without delay.

Communication is also vital even as a lone worker. I keep the relevant clinical teams informed when urgent results are delayed due to workload and escalate any unexpected issues to senior staff if required. Documentation is vital in demonstrating attention to detail, as any deviation or incident must be traceable and compliant with ISO15189 and internal SOPs.

Working as a lone scientist also improves my problem-solving and decision-making skills, as I learn to independently troubleshoot analysers, verify results, and manage multiple tasks under pressure. For example, I once managed a late-night situation where a biochemistry analyser flagged multiple patient samples as requiring repeat analysis due to interference. I prioritised the critical results, re-analysed urgent samples, and documented the deviations before notifying the on-call consultant - all while maintaining standard procedures and patient safety.

Summary:

As a lone worker in a high-pressure environment, I cope by planning and prioritising my tasks, multitasking efficiently, maintaining careful attention to detail, and communicating effectively with clinical teams. Across biochemistry, haematology, and microbiology, I ensure that all urgent and routine samples are processed accurately and according to SOPs. This approach allows me to maintain high laboratory standards and patient safety, while also developing my independence, problem-solving, and decision-making skills.

Question 56:

Why do you take temperature reading in the lab?

Background:

Laboratory materials such as reagents, calibrators, and control samples must be stored under the correct temperature conditions. Maintaining the correct storage conditions is vital for preserving the stability, potency, and reliability of laboratory materials, including reagents, calibrators, and control samples, to ensure accurate and dependable results. If these conditions are not upheld, reagents may deteriorate, compromising both analytical accuracy and patient safety. Similarly, recommended laboratory ambient temperatures are important to protect staff wellbeing and ensure that equipment functions optimally. Following these practices aligns with ISO 15189 standards and broader quality assurance requirements. This question is designed to test your understanding of the critical importance of cold chains and temperature monitoring in pathology laboratories. .

Points to consider:

- Importance of cold chain management.

- Laboratory recommended temperatures in line with ISO15189.
- Impact of out-of-range temperatures on materials, reagents, and equipment.
- Use practical examples where applicable.

Answer:

Taking temperature readings in the laboratory is a vital quality assurance measure to ensure both materials and equipment remain within the manufacturer's recommended ranges. These readings help identify when conditions deviate from set limits, allowing timely intervention to protect reagent stability, staff safety, and equipment performance.

For example, in biochemistry, reagents and calibrators stored in fridges at 2–8 °C can lose potency if exposed to fluctuating temperatures, potentially leading to inaccurate patient results. In blood transfusion, blood components are highly temperature dependent: red cells must be stored at 2–6 °C, while platelets require storage at 20–24 °C with agitation. Any deviation from these conditions could render the products unsafe for transfusion. In microbiology, agar plates stored at excessively warm temperatures may dry out and lose their diagnostic selectivity.

If I find a temperature reading out of range, I will quarantine the affected materials, record the incident, and escalate to my senior or manager for further investigation. This ensures patient safety is not compromised, and any affected samples are not used until confirmed safe.

Summary:

I take temperature readings in the laboratory to ensure quality assurance, patient safety, and staff wellbeing. This practice helps to maintain reagents, consumables, and equipment within the ranges recommended by ISO 15189. For example, in blood transfusion, red cells stored outside 2–6 °C could be unsafe for use, while in microbiology, agar plates stored at excessively warm temperatures may lose diagnostic

selectivity. If readings fall outside the acceptable range, I would quarantine the affected materials and escalate the issue for investigation, ensuring that no unsafe materials are used for patient testing.

Question 57:

A time you worked in a team, and it was not favourable

Background:

Pathology laboratories, like other areas in healthcare, attract people from different cultural and professional backgrounds. While teamwork is vital to maintaining high standards and ensuring patient safety, differences in opinion, working style, or communication can sometimes lead to tension. The key is to remain focused on the overall aim of the team: delivering safe, accurate, and timely results. This question is testing your understanding of how such challenges can affect teamwork and what action you can take to maintain standards, supported by practical examples.

Points to consider:

- Acknowledge possible differences between team members
- The importance of focusing on the shared goal
- Use communication and problem-solving skills
- Provide practical examples from pathology

Answer:

Teamwork is central to laboratory practice, but it can sometimes be challenging when differences arise. I experienced this while working on a particularly busy weekend in the haematology department, when we had a backlog of urgent full blood counts and coagulation samples. One colleague wanted to prioritise routine samples first, while I and another team member felt the urgent ITU and A&E requests should be processed before routine work. The disagreement led to some tension within the team.

To resolve this, I calmly reminded the team of the SOP guidance and ISO 15189 principles, which state that urgent and critical samples must always take priority. I then proposed dividing the workload: one person would focus on clearing urgent requests, while the others addressed the backlog of routine samples. This approach ensured that patient safety was maintained while still making progress on the overall workload.

I have also seen similar situations in biochemistry, where differences in approach to troubleshooting a failed calibration caused friction. In that case, I encouraged open discussion, listened to each suggestion, and supported the team to agree on following the SOP step-by-step rather than personal preference.

Summary:

Working in a team is not always straightforward, but I have learned to stay calm, use good communication, and refocus the group on the overall aim of the team, which are maintaining patient safety and laboratory standards. Even in challenging situations, I try to be the voice that brings the team back to the agreed procedures and goals, ensuring that disagreements don't compromise quality or turnaround time.

Question 58:

How would you react to criticism/feedback?

Background:

It is natural to feel proud when you have contributed positively to patient care. However, sometimes things may not go as expected, perhaps due to an oversight or misjudgement. In those moments, it is equally natural to feel disappointed. The key is to respond constructively when feedback is given, even if it feels like criticism. This question is testing your understanding that things can go wrong in the laboratory, and that you must remain calm, professional, and focused on using feedback to improve.

Points to consider:

- Understanding the pathology laboratory environment
- Importance of feedback in improving competency
- Positive and calm approach to negative feedback
- Provide practical example

Answer:

Things may sometimes happen below the required standard, and this could lead to feedback that may feel like criticism. My approach is to take it as a learning curve rather than something personal. Feedback is one of the most effective ways to grow in competence, and this is consistent with ISO15189, which emphasises continuous improvement.

For example, in biochemistry, I once released a potassium result that had been flagged as haemolysed by a senior colleague. Initially, I felt disappointed, as I believed I had been thorough. However, rather than reacting defensively, I listened to the feedback, reviewed the SOP, and gained a clearer understanding of how haemolysis can falsely elevate potassium levels. This experience helped me to be more vigilant when handling haemolysed samples in the future.

Similarly, **in haematology,** during my early training I validated a full blood count without recognising abnormal scattergrams. My senior pointed it out, and although it initially felt like criticism, I took it as a chance to improve. I later spent more time reviewing abnormal cases and became more confident at identifying atypical scatter patterns.

Summary:

I react to criticism by embracing it as an opportunity to learn and improve. Feedback, whether positive or negative, is central to professional development in pathology. By staying calm, open-minded, and willing to reflect, I ensure that feedback strengthens my practice and ultimately improves the quality of service delivered to patients.

Question 59:

What is your greatest achievement and why?

Background:

Working in the pathology laboratory helps to contribute to patients' health and wellbeing, which in most cases can be considered an achievement. Sometimes, in order to contribute effectively, it requires undergoing additional training or developing new competencies. How this training supports your confidence and capability in contributing to patient care reflects professional growth. This question is asking about achievements that directly benefit the department or Trust, highlighting your professional development.

Points to consider:

- What you have learned to improve
- How the achievement supported your improvement
- Provide practical examples where applicable

Answer:

One of my greatest achievements in the laboratory has been successfully completing a specialist competency portfolio **in haematology**, which significantly enhanced my ability to contribute to patient care. Before this, I was competent in routine analysis but lacked confidence in interpreting complex coagulation profiles, such as monitoring anticoagulant therapy or identifying rare clotting factor deficiencies.

To achieve this, I undertook additional training, attended workshops, and sought mentorship from senior band 6 and band 7 biomedical scientists. Through this process, I developed the ability to troubleshoot analytical anomalies, interpret results more accurately, and validate complex cases in accordance with ISO 15189 standards. For example, during a case of suspected thrombophilia, I identified inconsistencies in the initial test results and repeated the testing correctly, ultimately ensuring an accurate patient diagnosis and timely intervention.

Another achievement was **in biochemistry**, where I participated in an internal quality assurance project to optimise sample processing workflow. I noticed delays in sample handling during peak hours, so I proposed a revised workflow for urgent and routine samples. After implementing the changes, we reduced turnaround time by 15% without compromising quality. This achievement not only improved patient care but also enhanced team efficiency and morale.

In microbiology, I contributed to a cross-departmental initiative to standardise culture identification protocols. By reviewing SOPs and coordinating training for junior staff, we reduced reporting errors and ensured consistent results across all shifts. This reinforced my understanding of the importance of teamwork and structured training in achieving departmental goals.

Summary:

My greatest achievement is developing specialised competencies and contributing to improvements in workflow and quality assurance across haematology, biochemistry, and microbiology. These achievements reflect my commitment to continual professional growth, improving patient care, and supporting the department's objectives. They demonstrate my ability to identify areas for improvement, implement practical solutions, and ensure that standards are consistently met, benefiting both patients and the laboratory team.

Question 60:

Do you consider yourself a leader or follower?

Background:

Pathology laboratories are highly collaborative environments where success depends on teamwork. Every team member brings strengths, and some naturally take on leadership roles while others are effective followers. Leaders often set the direction after consultations and ensure tasks are delegated appropriately, while followers execute these plans efficiently, ensuring standards are met. This question is testing your awareness of your working style and how it contributes to the overall success of the team.

Points to consider:

- Understanding that laboratory achievement is a team effort
- Recognising that both leaders and followers play vital roles in teamwork
- Awareness of your role and the strengths you bring to a team
- How you have developed leadership or followership skills over time
- Use practical examples from pathology departments

Answer:

I consider myself adaptable and able to function effectively both as a leader and as a follower, depending on the situation and the needs of the team. In pathology laboratories, the focus is always on patient safety and accurate results, so flexibility in my role is essential.

For example, in haematology, I led a small project to implement new QC procedures for an analyser. I coordinated team meetings, delegated tasks such as running control samples and documenting results, and ensured that deadlines were met while maintaining ISO 15189 standards. In this scenario, I demonstrated leadership by keeping the team focused and ensuring that the quality of work was not compromised.

Conversely, **in a biochemistry setting,** I act as a follower when a senior band 6 is leading the troubleshooting of a complex analyser issue. In this scenario, the senior provides direction on the steps to take. I support by performing the assigned tasks precisely, documenting results accurately, and ensuring that any suggested adjustments are carefully implemented. This allows the senior to manage the critical decisions while I contribute to the smooth resolution of the problem, maintaining workflow efficiency and patient safety.

I have also learned to develop leadership skills by observing senior colleagues, taking on small leadership responsibilities, and gaining confidence to lead when necessary. This dual ability allows me to contribute positively to the team's efficiency and ensure high standards of patient care are consistently achieved.

Summary:

I am both a leader and a follower, depending on the team's needs. I can lead projects and coordinate colleagues to meet quality standards, as seen in implementing new QC procedures, and I can effectively follow guidance in complex situations, such as analyser troubleshooting. This adaptability ensures the team achieves its goals efficiently while maintaining patient safety and laboratory standards.

Question 61:

What is your greatest strength and why?

Background:

The pathology laboratory thrives on teamwork, where each individual's strengths support the wider function of the department. While every staff member brings their own unique abilities, the most effective teams are those where one person's strengths help balance another's weaknesses. Recognising and articulating your own strength is important not only for self-awareness, but also for showing how you contribute to patient care, safety, and laboratory quality. This question is testing your understanding of the importance of strengths in teamwork, your awareness of what you personally bring to the table, and how that positively impacts laboratory standards.

Points to consider:

- Awareness of the importance of teamwork through individual strengths.
- Awareness of your personal strengths in a professional environment.
- How your strength contributes to patient safety, efficiency, and laboratory quality.
- Give practical examples where appropriate.
- Why this strength matters in a high-pressure clinical laboratory setting.

Answer:

I believe my greatest strength is attention to detail under pressure, which I have consistently found to be essential in the laboratory environment. The pathology laboratory is fast-paced and high-stakes, and even the smallest oversight can have significant consequences for patient safety. My ability to remain calm, focused, and thorough even when working under pressure has helped me ensure accurate and timely results.

For example, while working **in haematology** on a particularly busy night shift, I noticed a discrepancy between the analyser flag and the blood film findings. Instead of releasing the result immediately, I double-checked, prepared a manual blood film, and identified blasts that had not been clearly flagged. My attention to detail ensured the result was escalated urgently to the clinician, leading to the diagnosis of acute leukaemia. This reinforced to me how vital accuracy and detail are in maintaining patient safety.

In biochemistry, for example, I once received a very high potassium result from a sample. Before reporting it as a critical value, I repeated the analysis and carefully checked the sample integrity. On inspection, I noticed that the sample was haemolysed, meaning the red blood cells had broken down and released potassium into the plasma. By recognising this, I avoided reporting a falsely elevated result that could have led to unnecessary and potentially harmful treatment for the patient.

I also find this strength useful when supporting colleagues. For example, **in transfusion,** I once assisted a colleague who was under pressure with an urgent crossmatch request. By carefully checking the patient identifiers against the blood product and laboratory information system (LIS), I prevented what could have been a serious mismatch error. My ability to keep detail in focus while still being mindful of time helped the team deliver safe, urgent care to the patient.

Summary:

My greatest strength is my ability to maintain attention to detail under pressure. I believe this is critical in pathology, where even a small oversight can affect patient safety. This strength has allowed me to identify potential errors in haematology blood films, prevent misreporting of biochemistry results during downtime, and support safe transfusion practices under time pressure. I see this not only as a personal strength, but also as a contribution to the wider team effort, because it helps uphold laboratory quality and patient safety even in high-pressure situations.

Question 62:

If you notice a non-conformity during an audit, what do you do?

Background:

Medical laboratories are ideally accredited according to the requirements of ISO15189, meaning that any action not consistent with the standards is considered a non-conformance. When it comes to audits whether internal or external are used to assess compliance or conformance, highlight non-conformance, and identify areas for improvement. When a non-conformance is identified, it must be reported, investigated, and documented. Root cause analysis ensures that corrective or preventive actions can be implemented to prevent recurrence. This question is testing your understanding of the role of audit, the importance of reporting non-conformance, and how it leads to continuous laboratory quality improvement.

Points to consider:

- What non-conformance is and why escalation is needed for quality improvement
- The role of audit in improving laboratory quality in line with ISO15189
- Give practical examples

Answer:

Non-conformance is any action, process, or outcome that does not comply with the laboratory's SOPs, ISO15189 requirements, or internal quality systems. If I notice a non-conformance during an audit, my first step would be to document it clearly, referencing the exact standard or SOP it relates to. I would then escalate it to the quality manager or senior staff, ensuring it is formally recorded, usually through an incident or non-conformance report form.

It is important not to assign blame, but instead to focus on identifying the root cause. For example, was the non-conformance due to inadequate training, equipment failure, unclear SOPs, or human error? Conducting this investigation is vital, as it helps prevent recurrence and contributes to overall quality improvement.

Practical examples:

Haematology: During an internal audit, I once noticed that a staff member had processed a blood film without completing the mandatory checklist for critical smear reviews. This was logged as a non-conformance, retraining was provided, and the checklist was reinforced in team meetings to prevent oversight.

Biochemistry: An audit highlighted that temperature logs for a fridge storing reagents were incomplete. I reported it, and after root cause analysis, we introduced automated temperature monitoring and alerts to strengthen compliance.

Transfusion: During a UKAS audit, a discrepancy was noted in the traceability records for blood units. By raising it immediately, the team was able to reconcile records and implement a double-check procedure before final sign-off, ensuring compliance with MHRA and ISO standards.

Summary:

If I notice a non-conformance during an audit, I will document it, escalate it, and ensure root cause analysis is carried out. The focus is on system improvement rather than fault-finding. For example, in biochemistry, I reported incomplete temperature logs, which led to the introduction of automated monitoring. This demonstrates my awareness that reporting non-conformance is not just about compliance only, but it is about improving patient safety, strengthening laboratory processes, and ensuring continual alignment with ISO15189 standards.

Question 63:

If a sample goes missing after receiving in the pathology lab, what do you do?

Background:

Laboratories receive large volumes of samples every day, and while sample misplacement is uncommon, it can occur due to human error or technical issues. For example, a sample could get trapped in an analyser, be left in a sample pod, or incorrectly logged in the system. Missing samples can have serious consequences, especially if they are urgent or relate to patient treatment, diagnosis, or emergencies. Such incidents should always be investigated thoroughly to identify the root cause and implement measures to prevent recurrence. This question is testing your understanding of the impact of missing samples on patient care and your approach to investigating and mitigating such events.

Points to consider:

- Impact of missing samples on patients
- Importance of investigating missing samples and implementing measures to reduce recurrence
- Proactive checking of outstanding results to identify unprocessed or misplaced samples
- Communicating with wards or clinicians to explain the situation and request a repeat sample
- Reporting the incident according to laboratory protocol
- Provide practical examples

Answer:

If I discover a sample is missing, my **first priority** is to understand the potential impact on the patient. For example, if the sample is from an urgent ward such as A&E, ITU, or the delivery suite, any delay could directly affect patient care. I would immediately check the laboratory information system and any outstanding sample lists to verify that the sample was indeed received and logged.

Next, I would physically search common areas, including analysers, centrifuges, storage fridges, and workbenches, as technical or procedural errors sometimes result in samples being misplaced temporarily. **In a biochemistry setting**, for instance, a sample could be left in a centrifuge rotor after spinning, or in a sample rack awaiting analysis. **In haematology**, a sample could be trapped in the barcode reader or in a storage rack due to misalignment.

Once a sample is confirmed missing, I would promptly contact the requesting ward or clinician, explain the situation, and request a repeat sample to ensure patient care is not compromised. I would document the missing sample, including times, locations checked, and actions taken, and report it formally as an incident in accordance with the laboratory's SOP and ISO 15189 quality management procedures.

Finally, I would reflect on how the sample went missing and discuss with the team to implement preventive measures. For example, retraining staff on proper sample handling, reinforcing the double-check system during logging, or after the incident, I reviewed the analyser maintenance procedures to ensure that all steps were being consistently followed. This included checking that the sample trays and rotors were correctly cleaned and cleared after each run, that routine calibration and preventive maintenance were up to date, and that staff were following the SOP for unloading samples. By reinforcing these procedures, the likelihood of samples being trapped, misplaced, or overlooked in the analyser is significantly reduced, helping to prevent similar incidents in the future.

Scenario-based Answer:

In a previous role, I noticed that a potassium sample from the A&E ward was not showing on our system. My first step was to check the outstanding samples list and the analyser logs to see if it had been processed or mis logged. After not finding it there, I physically checked the centrifuge, sample racks, and storage fridges. While searching, I reminded myself that in biochemistry, samples can occasionally be left in the rotor, and in haematology, tubes can sometimes get stuck in storage racks.

Once I confirmed the sample was missing, I immediately phoned the A&E ward, explained the situation, and requested a repeat sample to prevent any delay in patient management. I documented all steps, escalated the incident to my senior, and we reviewed the laboratory processes. As a result, we reinforced the double-check system at sample reception and implemented a reminder to ensure analysers are checked for residual tubes at the end of each run.

This approach ensured patient safety was maintained, the incident was properly reported, and measures were put in place to reduce the risk of recurrence.

Summary:

If a sample goes missing, my focus is always on patient safety first. I would proactively search and investigate the sample's whereabouts, communicate clearly with clinical teams to prevent delays in patient care, and formally report the incident

for quality improvement. By taking these steps, I ensure that patient wellbeing is protected, laboratory standards are maintained, and any systemic issues that contributed to the incident are addressed to prevent recurrence.

Question 64:

Do you have any question for us?

Background:

The interview panel will often give candidates the opportunity to ask questions at the end. It is not ideal to respond with "I don't have any questions," as this could suggest a lack of interest in the role or limited research about the Trust. Asking questions demonstrates enthusiasm, initiative, and genuine interest in the position and the organisation. This question is testing what you know about the Trust, whether you have considered aspects of the role that may be unclear, and your engagement as a potential staff member.

Points to consider:

- Show enthusiasm about working with the Trust.
- Ask questions based on your research or observations about the Trust.
- Inquire about aspects such as working patterns, CPD, professional development, or team collaboration.
- Focus on questions that demonstrate your desire to contribute to service improvement and patient care.

Answer

At the end of the interview, I would recommend that you ask thoughtful questions to demonstrate enthusiasm and interest in the Trust. For example, you could ask about opportunities for continuing professional development within the laboratory, such as training for specialist techniques or support for achieving higher band roles like completing your specialist portfolio. You can also inquire about staff wellbeing initiatives, particularly during high-pressure periods or out-of-hours shifts, and how the teams collaborate across different pathology departments.

You could ask about the introduction of new technologies or automation in the laboratory, and how staff are involved in adopting these changes, which demonstrates your interest in service improvement and professional development. It is also useful to ask when you can expect to hear from them, as this shows your enthusiasm for joining the team.

Practical example:

During my research about the Trust, I noticed the laboratory participates in several quality improvement initiatives. You might ask how staff are engaged in these initiatives or whether there are opportunities to contribute ideas for process improvements. This demonstrates both enthusiasm and an understanding of the importance of continual improvement in laboratory services.

Summary:

Thank you. Please, I would like to know more about the support available for completing a specialist portfolio, how out-of-hours working patterns are managed, and how staff are involved in quality improvement initiatives. I am keen to contribute to the team, maintain high standards, and continue developing my skills as a biomedical scientist. Also, could you let me know when I should expect to hear back regarding the outcome of this interview?

Question 65:

Would you perform a test on expired reagents (no other reagent available)?

Background:

The potency or viability of reagents can be affected by expiration or improper storage. Using expired reagents may lead to inaccurate results, which could impact patient diagnosis and treatment. ISO15189 and laboratory SOPs prohibit the use of expired reagents. This question is testing your understanding of reagent management, patient safety, and adherence to laboratory quality standards.

Points to consider:

- Reagent potency in maintaining ISO15189 compliance.
- Checking reagent expiration dates
- Avoiding the use of expired reagents
- Following SOP and ISO15189 guidelines
- Practical examples of managing reagent availability and patient safety.

Answer:

I would not perform a test using an expired reagent under any circumstance, even if it is the only reagent available. Expired reagents can produce inaccurate results, potentially leading to incorrect clinical decisions and patient harm, which would be a non-conformance under ISO15189 standards.

The laboratory usually has a daily reagent check system in place, which helps identify reagents that are approaching expiration or running low. Once identified, the SOP recommends ordering a new reagent to arrive before the current stock expires or runs out. Failure to follow this process, resulting in reagent expiration without any alternatives, would be considered a non-conformance and should be investigated and primary root cause identified. This may result to SOP update or change in policies to prevent recurrence.

Before introducing a new reagent into use, I would verify and validate it according to laboratory procedures to ensure it is ready for testing. This ensures no delay in turnaround time (TAT) and supports patient safety and wellbeing.

If a reagent is about to expire or unexpectedly runs out, I would proactively contact another site within the Trust to supply the reagent. If that is not possible, I would arrange for the sample to be processed at a nearby hospital and request that the hospital phones the result through. I would then document the results in the patient's LIMS, noting where the sample was processed and who communicated the result. Expired reagents would be safely discarded in the designated biohazard or chemical waste bin according to SOP. This approach ensures patient safety, maintains compliance with the quality management system, and minimizes disruption to service.

Summary:

Thank you. I would never use an expired reagent, as it could compromise patient safety. I would use the laboratory's daily reagent checks to anticipate expiration and order replacements proactively. If reagents run out unexpectedly, I would coordinate with another Trust site or a nearby hospital to ensure testing continues without delay. Expired reagents would be safely discarded following SOPs. This ensuring compliance and patient safety at all times.

Question 66:

Your colleague is making a mistake on bench, what would you do? Would you tell the senior or manager about it?

Background:

While mistakes are inevitable in the laboratory, it is essential that work is only carried out by staff who are trained and competent in the task. Both ISO 15189 and HCPC standards emphasise that staff should only undertake tasks in which they are confident and competent. Any observed mistake constitutes a non-conformance and should be investigated and escalated. This process helps maintain compliance with SOPs and regulatory requirements, while safeguarding patient safety and wellbeing. This question is designed to test your understanding of the impact of mistakes, patient safety, and non-compliance with UKAS ISO 15189 standards.

Points to consider:

- Recognise the impact of mistakes on laboratory quality and patient safety.
- Identify the mistake as a non-conformance that requires investigation.
- Correct the mistake directly if safe and appropriate.
- Report the issue directly to a senior or laboratory manager for further action.
- Provide practical examples from your experience.

Answer:

If I notice a mistake while a colleague is performing a task, I may alert them immediately, following the SOP, so the error can be corrected without affecting the sample or result. However, I would also inform the senior or laboratory manager, because alerting the colleague alone does not guarantee the mistake won't happen again. Reporting allows the senior to investigate the root cause and provide additional training or guidance if necessary.

For example:

Biochemistry: If a colleague is about to analyse a sample without proper centrifugation, I would pause the process and remind them of the requirement to centrifuge the sample correctly before analysis. I would still notify the senior or manager to ensure this oversight is addressed and does not recur.

Haematology: A colleague once ran a sample on the wrong analyser. I stopped the run immediately, corrected the process, and reported the incident to the senior scientist. The senior reviewed the SOP adherence and provided coaching to prevent similar errors.

Haematology / Phlebotomy: In another example, a colleague prepared a blood sample in the wrong anticoagulant tube. I intervened before analysis, corrected the issue, and informed the senior. The senior verified the sample, ensured corrective action was taken, and later used the incident as a teaching point in team training to prevent recurrence.

If I notice a mistake after the task is completed, I will first correct the issue safely and appropriately, then report it to the senior or manager to ensure the root cause is addressed and similar mistakes are prevented in the future.

Example:

In microbiology, a colleague once incubated a bacterial culture at the wrong temperature after completing the setup. I noticed this after the incubation had started, so I safely removed the plate, re-incubated it at the correct temperature, and documented the corrective action. I then reported the incident to the senior scientist, who investigated why the mistake occurred and reinforced proper temperature protocols with the team to prevent recurrence.

Summary:

Thank you. My approach is to ensure patient safety and laboratory quality by immediately correcting mistakes where possible, alerting the colleague during the process if necessary, and always informing the senior or manager so that the underlying causes can be investigated and addressed, ensuring compliance with ISO15189 and continuous improvement.

Question 67:

Please can you introduce yourself

Background:

This is one of the most common opening questions in an interview. It allows you to demonstrate your motivation for applying, your relevant academic and professional background, and the key experiences or skills you bring to the role. The focus is on how your journey and achievements align with the role you're interviewing for and with the Trust's values.

Points to consider:

- Mention your passion for the role and contribution to patient care.
- Outline academic and professional background.
- Highlight relevant experiences and competencies.
- Bring out transferable skills that add value to the team.
- Show alignment with NHS/Trust values (e.g., teamwork, compassion, equality, and quality).
- Use practical examples across pathology where possible.

Answer.

Thank you for the opportunity to introduce myself. My name is [X], and I am very passionate about working in pathology because it allows me to directly contribute to patient health and wellbeing by ensuring high-quality and accurate diagnostic results.

Academically, I hold a [mention your degree, e.g., BSc in Biomedical Science], and I am HCPC registered, which has equipped me with the theoretical knowledge and professional grounding required for this role. Over the course of my training and work placements, I have gained hands-on experience across multiple pathology disciplines, including haematology, biochemistry, and microbiology.

For example, in biochemistry, I have developed competence in operating and troubleshooting analysers, validating results, and maintaining quality assurance through daily internal QC and external QA schemes such as NEQAS. In haematology, I have experience running full blood counts, preparing blood smears, and validating abnormal results. In microbiology, I have supported specimen processing and culture identification, consistently adhering to SOPs and infection control protocols.

Alongside my technical skills, I bring strong teamwork, communication, and problem-solving abilities. For instance, during an out-of-hours lone shift in haematology, I managed a sudden influx of urgent samples by prioritising ITU and A&E requests, ensuring critical results were delivered on time while keeping to quality standards.

I also value professional growth and continuous development. I have actively participated in audits and quality improvement discussions, and I am particularly interested in supporting specialist portfolio development and CPD activities within the Trust.

Most importantly, I align with the Trust values of patient focus, inclusivity, and quality service. I see myself not just as a laboratory scientist but as someone committed to ensuring safe, reliable, and timely diagnostics that ultimately impact patient outcomes.

Summary:

Thank you. In summary, I am a passionate and motivated biomedical scientist with strong academic training, hands-on experience across multiple pathology departments, and a commitment to teamwork and patient safety. I believe my technical skills, problem-solving ability, and alignment with the Trust's values make me well-suited for this role, and I am excited about the opportunity to contribute positively to your team and to patient care.

Question 68:

Tell us the challenges you have faced in the laboratory

Background:

Biomedical Scientists and pathology laboratory staff often encounter challenges such as high workloads, equipment breakdown, staff shortages, or sample quality issues. These challenges can place pressure on turnaround times (TAT) and staff performance. However, laboratories accredited under ISO15189 expect staff to manage these issues effectively without compromising patient safety or laboratory quality. This question is testing your ability to acknowledge challenges, manage them appropriately, and stay focused on the overall laboratory quality and patient wellbeing.

Points to consider:

- Common challenges in pathology labs (workload, IT/system failure, equipment downtime, staff shortages, urgent samples).
- How to manage them while maintaining quality and TAT.
- Importance of teamwork, prioritisation, and communication.
- Giving practical example.
- Showing that challenges are seen as learning opportunities.

Answer:

Challenges are an inevitable part of working in a pathology laboratory, especially in a 24/7 environment, but the key is how you manage them without compromising patient safety.

One common challenge I have faced is high workload during staff shortages. For example, **in haematology,** when a colleague called in sick unexpectedly during a night shift, I was the only BMS covering urgent A&E and ITU samples. I used my prioritisation skills to focus on emergency samples first, such as blood films for suspected malaria and urgent full blood counts, before moving on to routine work. By maintaining communication with clinical staff, I was able to set realistic expectations while still ensuring critical results were delivered on time.

Another challenge I have experienced is analyser breakdown. **In biochemistry,** one of our analysers failed during a busy morning shift with a backlog of samples already coming from A&E. I quickly followed the SOP, placed the analyser into downtime mode, and transferred urgent samples to a backup analyser. For less urgent tests, I contacted a nearby site within the Trust to assist with processing. This not only ensured service continuity but also minimised disruption to patient care.

In blood transfusion, I once faced a situation where a patient required an urgent crossmatch, but the sample received was haemolysed. This was challenging because delaying a blood transfusion could have serious consequences. I immediately contacted the ward, explained the situation, and arranged for a repeat sample while preparing group O emergency blood as a backup option in case the patient's condition worsened. This approach ensured patient safety while maintaining compliance with laboratory policy.

Another common challenge is IT system downtime. During one shift, the LIMS went down, preventing the electronic release of results. Following the SOP, I manually recorded the results, communicated critical values directly to the wards, and later updated the LIMS once the system was restored. This ensured that patient management was not delayed despite the IT failure.

These challenges have taught me the importance of planning, prioritisation, communication, and teamwork, as well as maintaining composure under pressure to protect both patient safety and laboratory standards.

Summary:

I have faced several challenges in the laboratory, such as staff shortages, analyser breakdown, and IT downtime. For example, in haematology during a night shift, I was the only BMS covering urgent samples, and I had to carefully prioritise A&E and ITU work first. In biochemistry, I dealt with an analyser failure by transferring urgent tests to a backup analyser and contacting another site for support. And in blood transfusion, I managed an urgent case by arranging for a repeat sample while preparing emergency group O blood as a precaution.

In all these situations, I stayed calm, followed SOPs, communicated clearly with clinical teams, and ensured patient safety remained the top priority. I see challenges not just as difficulties but also as opportunities to improve my problem-solving, teamwork, and resilience.

Question 69:

What would you like to change in the lab?

Background:

In any pathology laboratory, there are always opportunities for improvement, whether in workflow efficiency, staff support, communication, or technology. When asked this question, it's important to avoid sounding overly critical. Instead, focus on constructive suggestions that align with patient safety, quality improvement, and staff development. This shows passion for care and a proactive mindset toward service improvement.

Points to consider:

- Show that your suggestion is linked to improving patient outcomes, staff wellbeing, or efficiency.
- Provide realistic, constructive ideas rather than complaints.
- Demonstrate that you are already thinking like part of the team, keen to make positive contributions.
- Use practical examples to support your answer

Answer:

If I had the opportunity to change something in the laboratory, I would focus on improving communication and feedback mechanisms between staff and senior management. While SOPs and guidelines provide clear direction, sometimes day-to-day challenges such as equipment downtime or workload surges can leave staff feeling under pressure. Creating a stronger system where staff can give quick feedback, and management can act on it, would improve both workflow efficiency and morale.

For example, **in biochemistry,** I have observed that when analysers go down during busy periods, staff sometimes spend extra time troubleshooting individually before escalating the issue. If there was a structured escalation system with quicker access to senior support, we could reduce downtime and ensure patients' urgent samples are processed without delay.

Another area I would like to change is the stock management system. In one instance **in haematology,** reagents ran critically low, creating pressure on staff to request emergency support from another site. Introducing a more automated stock alert system, integrated with LIMS, could help prevent this by flagging stock levels earlier, ensuring uninterrupted service and protecting turnaround times.

In microbiology, I believe investment in further automation could also be transformative. Routine plate reading, for example, can be time-consuming, and introducing automated culture analysers could free staff to focus on more complex interpretative work, improving efficiency and diagnostic accuracy.

Summary:

Thank you. If given the opportunity, I would like to see improvements in areas that directly impact both staff and patients. For example, strengthening communication and escalation processes during equipment downtime, improving stock management with automated alerts, and supporting investment in automation in microbiology. These changes would reduce unnecessary delays, improve staff efficiency, and most importantly, enhance patient safety and wellbeing.

Question 70:

What do you do when you receive a new machine in the lab?

Background:

According to ISO15189, any new equipment, analyser, or reagent must be verified and validated before being brought into routine use. This ensures the instrument performs according to the manufacturer's specifications and meets the laboratory's quality standards. The process includes maintenance checks, calibration, QC, validation, documentation, and staff training. Measurement of uncertainty (MU) is also part of validation to demonstrate the reliability of reported results.

Points to consider:

- Equipment installation, verification, and validation before clinical use.
- Preventive maintenance and calibration.
- Quality Control (QC) testing across all levels.
- Correlation studies with existing analysers.
- Measurement of Uncertainty (MU).
- SOP development, documentation, and staff training.
- Practical examples where applicable.

Answer:

When a new analyser arrives in the laboratory, I would follow the verification and validation process in line with ISO15189 and the laboratory's SOPs before using it for patient samples. This involves several steps:

Maintenance Checks: I would first ensure that the analyser undergoes preventive maintenance and safety checks, confirming it is in good working condition before calibration.

Calibration: Once maintenance is complete, the analyser would be calibrated according to the manufacturer's requirements to establish baseline accuracy.

Quality Control (QC) Testing: Internal QC would be run across abnormal low, normal, and abnormal high ranges to confirm precision and reproducibility.

Correlation Studies: Patient samples would be tested on both the new and existing analysers, and results compared to confirm equivalence.

Measurement of Uncertainty (MU): During validation, I would calculate MU using QC data and repeated measurements to understand the degree of variability in results. This is important for clinical decision making. For example, if a potassium result is reported as 5.0 mmol/L ± 0.2, the clinician knows the **"true"** value is likely between 4.8-5.2 mmol/L. This helps prevent misinterpretation, especially around critical cut-offs.

SOP Development/Update: After validation, I would update or create SOPs to document analyser use, QC, calibration, troubleshooting, and MU reporting.

Staff Training and Competency: I would ensure all staff are trained on the analyser and updated SOP, and that competency is assessed before routine use begins.

Practical Example (Biochemistry):

When we validated a new biochemistry analyser, we carried out full QC across all levels and compared results with the old analyser. For potassium, we calculated the MU as ±0.2 mmol/L. This was important because potassium is critical in emergency care - ensuring that even at decision thresholds (e.g., 6.0 mmol/L), clinicians had confidence in the accuracy of the result. The MU, along with calibration and validation records, was documented in the SOP, and all staff were trained before patient testing began.

Practical Example (Haematology):

When a new FBC analyser was introduced, we validated it by running duplicate patient samples and comparing them with the old analyser. MU was also calculated for haemoglobin and platelet counts to assess reliability. The validation data was documented, and staff were trained on the updated SOP before the analyser was used on patient samples.

Summary:

If I receive a new machine in the laboratory, I ensure it undergoes installation and full maintenance checks, followed by calibration, QC testing, correlation with existing analysers using known patient samples, and measurement of uncertainty as part of validation. I would then support the development or updating of the SOP before staff training and competency assessments are carried out. For example, in biochemistry, I was involved in validating a new analyser by checking maintenance, calibration, running QC at all levels, and comparing patient results, such as sodium and creatinine, with the existing analyser. Only once all these

steps were completed and documented was the analyser released for routine patient testing. This approach ensures compliance with ISO 15189, maintains patient safety, and supports service continuity.

Question 71:

How do you train Band 5 scientists in your lab?

Background:

Training in the pathology laboratory is a crucial process to ensure staff competence, standardisation, and consistency in laboratory performance. While a Band 5 Biomedical Scientist is often newly qualified, some may already have significant experience. The aim of training is to ensure that all staff are competent and confident in carrying out assigned tasks in accordance with ISO 15189, the SOPs, and the laboratory's quality management system (QMS). This question is designed to test your understanding of how to structure, deliver, and assess training effectively to ensure competency and maintain service quality.

Points to consider:

- Importance of structured training and competency assessment
- Understanding that training is both technical and organisational (orientation and integration)
- Following ISO 15189 and QMS for competency sign-off
- Role of supervision, mentorship, and feedback
- Use of practical examples to support your answer.

Answer:

Training a Band 5 Biomedical Scientist requires a structured approach that balances technical competence with integration into the laboratory culture. I begin by ensuring that the staff member is welcomed and oriented to the working environment. For example, I would take them around the laboratory, introduce them to colleagues, and show them key facilities such as the staff room, canteen, and locker areas. This initial step helps new staff feel comfortable and included a vital foundation for effective learning.

Once settled, I ensure the staff member has access to Q-Pulse (or an equivalent QMS platform), where I allocate relevant SOPs, health and safety guidelines, and laboratory policies. This helps them understand laboratory expectations, procedures, and standards before hands-on training begins. I encourage them to ask questions and clarify any doubts, ensuring they develop a solid understanding of the theoretical aspects of their role.

For bench training, I adopt a "train-by-example" approach. I demonstrate the correct technique or process. For instance, preparing samples, loading analysers, or validating results while explaining each step and the rationale behind it. In biochemistry, this might involve demonstrating correct pipetting techniques and analyser calibration; in haematology, running and interpreting daily quality control (QC) results; or in microbiology, correct plate inoculation and incubation procedures.

As their confidence develops, I allow staff to perform tasks under supervision, providing real-time feedback and correction. For example, when validating results in haematology, I observe their process and discuss their reasoning for any flagged results. Once consistent competence is demonstrated, I allow the staff member to work independently while continuing to review and validate their work before final sign-off.

When both the trainee and I are satisfied with their performance, I initiate competency assessment in line with ISO 15189 standards. This includes written or practical assessments, followed by documentation and sign-off confirming their readiness to work independently. If gaps are identified, I provide targeted retraining to ensure they fully meet laboratory standards before final authorisation.

Summary:

I believe effective training combines structured orientation, demonstration, supervision, feedback, and formal competency assessment. For instance, when I trained a Band 5 colleague in biochemistry, I first introduced them to the lab systems and SOPs, demonstrated daily analyser maintenance and QC, then gradually allowed them to perform independent analysis. Once they consistently produced accurate results and demonstrated full understanding, I completed their competency sign-off. This approach ensures quality, consistency, and confidence supporting both the staff member's development and the laboratory's ISO 15189 commitment to maintaining a competent workforce.

Question 72:

What do you do when your EQA report comes back below expected required standard?

Background:

External Quality Assessment (EQA) schemes are a vital part of maintaining high laboratory standards and ensuring the accuracy and reliability of results. EQA enables laboratories to compare their performance with other participating labs and identify analytical or procedural errors that may not be detected through internal quality control (IQC) alone. A below-standard EQA result indicates a potential issue that must be investigated and corrected promptly to maintain ISO 15189 compliance, safeguard patient safety, and uphold confidence in laboratory results.

Points to consider:

- Understanding what an EQA scheme is and its purpose in quality assurance.
- Importance of consistent participation in EQA schemes to monitor accuracy and inter-laboratory comparability.

- Potential causes of poor EQA performance (e.g., calibration drift, reagent deterioration, analyser malfunction, or human error).
- Steps to investigate poor EQA performance - review of IQC trends, repeat testing, equipment checks, staff competency review.
- Implementation of corrective and preventive actions (CAPA) and proper documentation in accordance with ISO15189.
- Give practical examples to support answer

Answer:

If an EQA report returns below the expected performance standard, I would first treat it as a non-conformance and begin a structured investigation in line with the laboratory's SOP and ISO15189 quality management system.

The first step would be to review the EQA report in detail. For example, identifying the specific analyte or parameter that failed and the type of error (systematic or random). I would then check recent internal quality control (IQC) trends for the same parameter to see if there has been any drift, bias, or instability leading up to the EQA distribution.

Next, I would repeat the EQA sample (if still available) alongside IQC material and fresh patient samples to confirm whether the issue persists. If the repeat result remains outside the acceptable range, I would escalate the issue to the senior BMS or section lead to begin a deeper investigation.

The next stage would include:

- Reviewing calibration and maintenance records of the analyser to ensure calibration was up to date and preventive maintenance was performed correctly.

- Checking reagent lot numbers and expiry dates to ensure they were valid and consistent with those used at the timo of EQA testing.

- Assessing staff competency, particularly if a new or unfamiliar user performed the original test.
- Examining pre-analytical and post-analytical factors, such as sample handling, incorrect pipetting, or data transcription errors.

Once the root cause is identified, I would implement corrective actions (e.g., recalibration, staff retraining, or reagent replacement) and document everything in the non-conformance or EQA corrective action log. I would also monitor subsequent EQA and IQC performance to ensure the issue does not recur - this forms the preventive action and supports continual improvement.

Practical Examples:

Biochemistry: If potassium EQA returned outside limits, I would check whether a new reagent lot was introduced and verify if calibration drift occurred. Once, our lab noticed a consistent negative bias on sodium results in EQA - investigation revealed that the ion-selective electrode required cleaning and recalibration. After corrective action, both IQC and EQA performance normalised.

Haematology: In one instance, the EQA for haemoglobin showed a low bias. Review of the analyser logs showed a calibration issue after reagent change. After recalibration and verification, subsequent EQA performance improved.

Transfusion: If EQA for antibody screening showed an unexpected result, I would review reagent cell expiry and ensure all staff involved in reading the panels had up-to-date competency.

Summary:

If an EQA result returned below standard, I would address it systematically by reviewing IQC trends, calibration, reagents, and staff performance in accordance with ISO 15189 and the SOP. I would document the non-conformance, carry out a root-cause analysis, and implement corrective and preventive measures.

For example, in biochemistry, when an EQA showed a negative bias for sodium, I led the investigation that identified a calibration issue. After recalibration and verification, both IQC and EQA results returned to expected performance. This experience reinforced the importance of maintaining a strong internal quality system and proactive communication with senior staff to uphold patient safety and service quality.

Question 73:

Discuss QMS in the lab?

Background:

A Quality Management System (QMS) ensures that all activities in the pathology laboratory are carried out in a controlled, consistent, and traceable manner to guarantee reliable patient results. It provides the structure that ensures quality (meeting expected standards) and management (the systems and processes) work together to deliver accurate, timely, and safe laboratory services.

Under ISO15189, the QMS is built around 12 Quality System Essentials (QSEs), which serve as pillars for achieving and maintaining accreditation. These essentials ensure that every part of laboratory operations from staff competency to equipment maintenance contributes to continual improvement and patient safety.

Points to consider:

- What QMS means and its purpose in the laboratory
- The 12 essentials of QMS and how they interlink
- The importance of QMS in achieving ISO15189 compliance
- Practical examples demonstrating QMS in action

Answer:

The Quality Management System (QMS) in the laboratory is a structured framework that integrates quality (meeting defined standards), management (coordinating and regulating processes), and system (the organised structure ensuring these are achieved). In simple terms, QMS ensures that every process in the laboratory from sample reception to result reporting is performed correctly, safely, and consistently to support patient care.

According to ISO15189, there are 12 Quality System Essentials (QSEs) that form the foundation of QMS:

1. **Organisation and Management** - Ensures a clear chain of command and responsibility. For example, laboratory managers oversee operations while quality officers ensure compliance.

2. **Personnel** - Staff must be trained, competent, and continually assessed. For example, BMSs complete competency assessments and CPD portfolios to remain current.

3. **Equipment** - All instruments must be maintained, calibrated, and verified before use. For example, daily analyser maintenance logs are checked before starting biochemistry runs.

4. **Purchasing and Inventory** - Ensures reagents and consumables are ordered, tracked, and stored properly. For example, reagents are logged into Q-Pulse and monitored for expiry.

5. **Process Control** - Covers all analytical procedures, from sample collection to result reporting. Internal Quality Control (IQC) ensures results are within acceptable limits before releasing patient results.

6. **Information Management** - Involves proper data handling and result entry via LIMS to ensure traceability and confidentiality.

7. **Documents and Records** - All procedures must have up-to-date SOPs, and records (like QC logs, maintenance records, and training files) must be easily retrievable.

8. **Occurrence Management** - Any non-conformance or incident (e.g., sample mislabelling) is reported, investigated, and corrective actions implemented.

9. **Assessment** - Regular internal and external audits assess compliance. For example, UKAS inspections verify that the lab meets ISO15189 requirements.

10. **Process Improvement** - Uses audit findings and staff feedback to improve services. For example, revising an SOP to simplify a complex process.

11. **Customer Service** - Ensures good communication with users such as clinicians and wards, responding to queries or complaints promptly.

12. **Facilities and Safety** - Focuses on ensuring a safe working environment, such as proper waste disposal, PPE use, and risk assessments.

Each of these elements is interconnected and contributes to the laboratory's continuous improvement and patient safety.

Practical Example:

In haematology, if a routine internal QC fails, the analyser is not used until the issue is resolved. The incident is documented under occurrence management, the analyser checked under equipment, and corrective actions recorded for process improvement. This demonstrates how QMS ensures issues are properly managed without compromising patient safety.

In biochemistry, QMS principles are followed through daily equipment checks, reagent lot validation, and EQA participation to ensure analytical accuracy.

In microbiology, QMS ensures that culture media batches are quality-checked before use, and results are verified by a competent scientist before release - aligning with process control and personnel essentials.

Summary:

My understanding of a Quality Management System (QMS) is that it provides a structured framework to ensure that every process in the laboratory meets expected standards, is well-managed, and continuously improved. It is built around the 12 Quality System Essentials of ISO 15189, which together safeguard patient safety, staff competence, and reliable results. For example, in biochemistry, if a QC fails, we do not simply fix it and move on. We document the incident, investigate the root cause, and implement corrective actions. This is QMS in action, ensuring consistency, accountability, and continuous improvement across all departments.

Question 74:

How do you ensure the right result is given to the right patient?

Background:

The pathology laboratory plays a critical role in patient diagnosis and treatment. Therefore, ensuring that the right result is issued to the right patient is central to patient safety and quality care. Errors can occur at any stage of sample collection to result reporting, which are pre-analytical, analytical, or post-analytical. Possible errors associated with any of these phases must be detected and corrected before results are released. This question tests understanding of laboratory structures and quality control processes that ensure result accuracy, reliability, and traceability.

Points to consider:

- Understanding what makes a result accurate and reliable.

- Measures in place across the pre-analytical, analytical, and post-analytical phases.
- How to identify and investigate non-compliance to improve systems.
- Importance of ISO15189, SOP adherence, and LIMS verification.
- Use of practical examples to demonstrate awareness.

Answer:

Ensuring the right result is given to the right patient requires maintaining accuracy, traceability, and reliability across all three phases of laboratory testing, which are: pre-analytical, analytical, and post-analytical. Each phase has built-in structures designed to detect, correct, and prevent errors that could lead to a wrong result being released.

Pre-Analytical Phase:

This is where most laboratory errors occur, often due to incorrect patient identification, mislabelling, wrong sample type, or poor sample quality. To minimise such errors, I ensure that each sample is correctly labelled with three identifiers (full name, date of birth, and hospital/NHS number), matching both the request form and the specimen. I also verify collection details on the LIMS before analysis. For example, **in haematology,** if a sample arrives clotted or with a mismatched label, I will reject the sample, document it in LIMS, and contact the ward to request a repeat sample, ensuring proper identification is verified before acceptance.

Analytical Phase:

At this stage, ensuring that equipment and methods are functioning correctly is essential for producing valid results. I verify that quality control (QC) is within acceptable limits before running patient samples, and if a QC fails, I do not proceed until the issue is resolved. I also check analyser flags, error codes, and result plausibility. For example, in biochemistry, if a patient's potassium result is extremely high but QC and analyser flags are normal, I examine the sample for haemolysis and compare it with previous results in the LIMS. If the result appears inconsistent, I repeat the test on a fresh aliquot before validation.

Post-Analytical Phase:

This phase ensures accurate result verification, validation, and communication. Before releasing results, I double-check that results are clinically and physiologically consistent. I compare them with the patient's historical data to identify unexpected trends. If results are critical or inconsistent, I contact the clinician or ward for clarification before authorising. For example, **in microbiology,** if a culture report identifies an unexpected organism inconsistent with the clinical information, I would discuss it with the senior BMS or consultant microbiologist before releasing the report.

Continuous Improvement:

If a result is found to have been incorrectly assigned, this would be treated as a non-conformance and reported through the laboratory's incident management system. A root cause analysis (RCA) would then be performed whether it was due to human error, system issue, or sample misidentification and corrective actions implemented, such as retraining or SOP updates.

Summary:

In summary, I ensure the right result is given to the right patient by adhering strictly to ISO 15189 standards, SOPs, and the three-phase laboratory process. I verify patient identifiers, ensure QC and analyser performance are within range, validate results before release, and communicate effectively with clinicians when necessary. For example, in biochemistry, I once detected an unusually high bilirubin in a neonate sample that appeared inconsistent with the clinical notes. I double-checked the sample ID, repeated the analysis, and confirmed it was a sample mix-up. I rejected the sample and cancelled the result, thereby preventing a potential misdiagnosis and ensuring patient safety.

Question 75:

Tell us when you made a mistake, how you corrected it, and what you learnt from the mistake.

Background:

The nature of pathology requires continuous learning and improvement. Mistakes, although undesirable, provide valuable opportunities for reflection, identifying areas for improvement, and enhancing competence. This question is testing your ability to recognise a mistake, correct it appropriately, and reflect on how it has contributed to your professional development.

Points to consider:

- Acknowledge the mistake honestly.
- Describe the immediate corrective actions taken to prevent patient impact.
- Demonstrate reflection and learning from the incident.
- Use practical examples (pre-analytical, analytical, post-analytical) to support your answer.

Answer:

During my work in the haematology department, I once mislabelled a sample tube during peak workload, which could have led to results being attributed to the wrong patient. Upon noticing the mistake during the initial check against the LIMS, I immediately isolated the sample and corrected the labelling according to the SOP. I then informed the senior scientist to ensure the incident was documented in the laboratory's non-conformance log.

In another instance in biochemistry, I once performed a sample analysis without checking the centrifugation status. The analyser flagged an abnormal result. I reviewed the sample, realised it had not been spun correctly, repeated the centrifugation, and re-ran the analysis. I then documented the incident and reflected on the need to consistently follow pre-analytical checks before analysis.

From these experiences, I have learnt the importance of vigilance at every stage of the laboratory process. I have also developed a habit of double-checking sample identity, labelling, and pre-analytical preparation before analysis. Additionally, I now share lessons learned during team huddles to help colleagues avoid similar mistakes. This approach has enhanced my attention to detail, reinforced adherence to SOPs, and strengthened overall laboratory quality.

Summary:

Thank you. One mistake I made was mislabelling a haematology sample. I corrected it immediately, informed my senior, and ensured proper documentation. In another case, I re-analysed a centrifugation error in biochemistry. These experiences taught me the importance of vigilance, following SOPs, and reflecting on incidents to prevent recurrence. I now proactively check and double-check all pre-analytical and analytical steps and share lessons with the team to maintain patient safety and laboratory quality.

Question 76:

How would you handle criticism on a job you didn't do well from a senior colleague?

Background:

In the pathology laboratory, receiving feedback or criticism especially from a senior colleague, is a normal part of professional growth. Mistakes or underperformance can occur due to workload pressure, unfamiliar procedures, or oversight. How one responds to constructive criticism reflects emotional intelligence, professionalism, and a genuine commitment to continuous improvement. This question evaluates your ability to remain composed, take responsibility, and learn from feedback, all while fostering positive working relationships. It also highlights your understanding that constructive criticism is an opportunity for growth, enhancing your skills and supporting patient safety.

Points to consider:

- Maintain professionalism and a calm, positive attitude.
- Accept responsibility and avoid being defensive.
- Reflect on what went wrong and how to prevent it next time.
- Seek clarification or retraining if needed.
- Demonstrate learning and improvement after the feedback.
- Use practical example to support your answer.

Answer:

Receiving constructive criticism from a senior colleague is part of professional development. My approach is to remain calm, listen carefully, and avoid being defensive. I would thank the senior colleague for the feedback, acknowledge any errors, and reflect on what led to the situation.

For example, **in biochemistry**, there was a time I mistakenly released a potassium result without noticing the analyser flag indicating a haemolysed sample. My senior colleague pointed it out, explaining that haemolysis can falsely elevate potassium levels. Instead of feeling discouraged, I saw it as an opportunity to improve. I reviewed the SOP on sample integrity, discussed analyser flags with the senior, and started double-checking all flagged results before validation. This experience strengthened my attention to detail and improved my understanding of pre-analytical errors.

Similarly, **in haematology,** if a senior colleague pointed out that I had not correctly followed the delta check policy for full blood counts, I would revisit the SOP, discuss the situation to clarify any confusion, and ensure I document my reflection for CPD purposes.

If I felt unclear about any part of the feedback, I would respectfully ask for guidance or further training. I believe that accepting feedback with humility and a willingness to learn helps build trust and fosters a culture of quality and improvement.

Summary:

If I received criticism from a senior colleague for a task I didn't perform well, I would listen attentively, remain calm, and view it as a constructive opportunity to improve. I would reflect on what went wrong, review relevant SOPs, and implement changes to prevent it happening again. For example, when I once missed an analyser flag in biochemistry, I learned to always check instrument alerts carefully before validating results. I see constructive feedback as a valuable way to grow professionally and contribute more effectively to maintaining high laboratory standards.

Question 77:

Discuss your last job description.

Background:

This question helps the panel understand your hands-on experience as a Biomedical Scientist and how your previous responsibilities align with the duties of the role you're applying for. It also gives you an opportunity to demonstrate how your practical, analytical, and quality management experience as well as any transferable skills gained from earlier roles support patient safety and laboratory efficiency in line with ISO 15189 standards.

Points to consider:

- Outline your key responsibilities as a Biomedical Scientist.
- Link your experience to ISO 15189, QMS, and SOP compliance.
- Include experiences across pre-analytical, analytical, and post-analytical stages.
- Demonstrate teamwork, problem-solving, and quality improvement involvement
- Use practical examples to show your contribution to service delivery.

Answer:

In my last role as a Biomedical Scientist, I was responsible for ensuring accurate, timely, and reliable analysis of patient samples across key pathology disciplines while maintaining compliance with ISO 15189 and the laboratory's Quality Management System (QMS). My day-to-day duties covered all three analytical phases, which are: pre-analytical, analytical, and post-analytical with a focus on patient safety and result accuracy.

During the pre-analytical phase, I verified that all samples were properly labelled and met acceptance criteria according to SOPs. For example, when I received a sample with a mismatched patient identifier, I immediately quarantined it, contacted the ward for clarification, and raised a non-conformance report through Q-Pulse. This ensured the right result was linked to the right patient while maintaining traceability and documentation standards.

In the analytical phase, I performed maintenance, calibration, and daily IQC checks on instruments such as the Sysmex XN analyser **in haematology** and the Roche Cobas 8000 **in biochemistry**. I ensured IQC and EQA results were within expected limits and investigated any outliers following the Westgard rules and manufacturer guidelines. For example, when I noticed a consistent QC drift in one biochemistry parameter, I stop testing, performed reagent replacement and recalibration, and escalated the issue to the senior BMS where applicable. This helped prevent the release of potentially inaccurate results and reinforced my understanding of analytical troubleshooting and documentation.

In the post-analytical phase, I validated and authorised results, ensuring they aligned with clinical expectations. For example, if a potassium result was critically high, I would review previous results, check for sample haemolysis, verify the date and time of sample collection, and consider potential EDTA contamination. I would also contact the ward to confirm the patient's status before authorising the result. This approach reflects my commitmont to both technical accuracy and clinical responsibility.

In addition to bench work, I was actively involved in training and mentoring Band 5 scientists and placement students, guiding them through SOPs, quality control procedures, and competency assessments. This experience developed my leadership and communication skills, allowing me to balance training responsibilities with daily workflow efficiency.

Before qualifying as a Biomedical Scientist, I also worked as a Medical Laboratory Assistant, where I developed an appreciation for pre-analytical quality from proper sample sorting to prioritising urgent requests. My earlier experience as a Healthcare Assistant further strengthened my understanding of patient care and sample integrity, which continues to guide my laboratory practice today.

Summary:

My last job as a Biomedical Scientist gave me comprehensive experience across all analytical phases, quality management, and training. I developed a strong understanding of ISO 15189 compliance, QMS documentation, and clinical relevance of laboratory results. My practical experience combined with my background as an MLA and Healthcare Assistant allows me to approach laboratory work with a holistic understanding of patient care. I believe these experiences have fully prepared me to contribute effectively to your team, ensuring high-quality results, excellent turnaround times, and continuous service improvement.

Question 78:

What are the quality measures to put in place at work?

Background:

In a pathology laboratory, quality measures are essential to ensure that all results produced are accurate, reliable, and reproducible, supporting safe and effective patient care. The ISO15189 standard defines the framework for maintaining quality in all laboratory processes from pre-analytical to post-analytical phases. These measures aim to minimise errors, promote consistency, and ensure continuous improvement. This question tests your understanding of how laboratory quality is maintained, monitored, and improved through quality measures.

Points to consider:

- Understanding of ISO15189 quality requirements.
- Importance of internal and external quality control.
- Use of SOPs, audits, documentation, and staff competency assessments.
- Importance of equipment maintenance and calibration.
- Regular training, CPD, and review of incidents/non-conformances.
- Use practical examples to support your answer

Answer:

Quality measures in the laboratory are structured systems and procedures designed to ensure that all analytical processes meet ISO15189 standards and support patient safety. These measures span the entire testing pathway from pre-analytical, analytical, and post-analytical.

In the **pre-analytical phase**, quality begins with proper sample collection, labelling, and transportation. For example, **in haematology**, ensuring that full blood count samples are collected in EDTA tubes and received within the required timeframe helps to avoid clotting or cell deterioration. The use of sample acceptance/rejection criteria and barcode verification ensures that only suitable samples are processed.

During the analytical phase, quality measures include daily internal quality control (IQC) checks, equipment calibration, and preventive maintenance. For example, in biochemistry, running IQC samples at low, normal, and high levels before patient testing ensures the analyser is performing accurately. Any QC failures are investigated immediately, and corrective actions are documented before continuing with patient work. Similarly, in microbiology, positive and negative control strains are tested alongside patient samples to verify test accuracy and reliability.

In the **post-analytical phase**, measures such as result validation, delta checks, and peer review ensure that ensure only accurate and clinically appropriate results are released. For example, when validating results in haematology, I cross-check abnormal results against previous results in LIMS to confirm consistency before authorising the report.

Beyond testing, quality is reinforced through training and competency assessments, SOP adherence, and document control systems like Q-Pulse, which ensure all staff are working to the most current standards. Regular audits help identify areas for improvement, and EQA participation benchmarks the laboratory's performance against other accredited labs.

When non-conformances occur, they are logged, investigated for root cause, and corrective/preventive actions (CAPA) are implemented. For example, if an EQA sample returns a poor result, a full investigation would be carried out to identify whether it was due to calibration error, reagent deterioration, operator error or any other forms of systematic (underlining) error.

Summary:

Quality measures at work encompass all the systems and procedures that maintain accuracy, reliability, and compliance with ISO15189. From pre-analytical checks, IQC/EQA participation, equipment calibration, and SOP adherence, to training and incident investigation. Every of these steps ensures patient safety and continuous service improvement. By consistently applying these quality measures, the laboratory builds confidence in the results it provides and contributes to high standards of patient care.

Question 79:

Describe how you have worked as a team.

Background:

Teamwork is central to the functioning of any pathology laboratory and the wider healthcare environment. Biomedical Scientists work closely with colleagues from different specialisms such as Haematology, Biochemistry, Microbiology, and Transfusion, as well as external healthcare teams like nurses and clinicians. A successful team relies on effective communication, respect for individual strengths, and shared responsibility for patient safety and timely service delivery. This question is testing your understanding of the importance of teamwork in achieving laboratory quality and your ability to demonstrate collaboration, communication, and professionalism through real examples.

Points to Consider:

- Understanding the importance of teamwork in delivering accurate and timely patient results.
- Acknowledging the diversity of team members and how their strengths complement each other.
- Demonstrating good communication and collaboration in different lab situations.
- Handling conflict or pressure in a professional way while maintaining focus on the patient.
- Use practical examples to support your answer.

Answer:

Teamwork is essential in the pathology laboratory because no one can deliver the full diagnostic service alone. Every result depends on coordinated effort from sample reception to analysis and final authorisation.

For example, **in Biochemistry,** I worked as part of a multidisciplinary team where effective communication and support were crucial during a particularly busy on-call shift. We had a surge in emergency samples, and one of our analysers went down.

Instead of panicking, we divided tasks. For example, one colleague focused on rerunning urgent samples on the backup analyser, while I communicated with the A&E ward to prioritise critical cases. This collaboration ensured minimal delay in turnaround time and avoided any negative impact on patient care.

Similarly, in Haematology, I collaborated with colleagues to troubleshoot inconsistent full blood count results. We reviewed possible causes and identified a calibration drift as the issue. Working together, one colleague recalibrated the analyser, another reviewed recent results, and I updated the senior staff on the incident, explaining how we restored accuracy and prevented the reporting of incorrect data.

Outside the lab, I also demonstrated teamwork when I worked as a Healthcare Assistant before qualifying as a Biomedical Scientist. I regularly collaborated with nurses and doctors to ensure patients received the right care, especially during ward rounds or blood collections. These experiences helped me appreciate the importance of communication, mutual respect, and understanding how laboratory results directly impact patient management.

Summary:

I believe teamwork is about mutual support, effective communication, and focusing on the shared goal of patient safety and quality service. For example, in Biochemistry, during a surge of emergency samples, I collaborated with colleagues to rerun urgent tests on a backup analyser while communicating with A&E to prioritise critical cases, ensuring patient care was not compromised. In Haematology, I worked with colleagues to identify a calibration drift affecting full blood count results, coordinating tasks to correct the issue and prevent incorrect reporting.

Even in my previous role as a Healthcare Assistant, I worked closely with nurses and doctors during ward rounds to ensure accurate blood collections and timely patient care. These experiences taught me that clear communication, respect for colleagues' expertise, and effective teamwork under pressure

are essential for delivering consistent, high-quality results and supporting the overall healthcare service.

Question 80:

You have a staff making mistake at work, how will you help the staff.

Background:

In a pathology laboratory, mistakes can occur despite training and competency. Supporting a colleague when they make a mistake is essential to maintain patient safety, laboratory quality, and team morale. ISO15189 emphasizes that non-conformances should be identified, corrected, and used as learning opportunities. This question is testing your understanding of how to correct mistakes constructively, provide support, and prevent recurrence.

Points to consider:

- Understanding the impact of mistakes on patient safety and laboratory quality
- Correcting the mistake promptly and safely
- Providing guidance or coaching to the staff member
- Reporting to senior or manager where necessary
- Using practical examples to support your answer

Answer:

If I notice a staff member making a mistake, my approach is first to ensure patient safety and laboratory quality are not compromised. I would intervene immediately if possible, and correct the error safely, following the SOP. After that, I would discuss the mistake with the staff member in a supportive way, explaining why the correct process is important and how to avoid similar errors in the future.

For example, **in biochemistry**, if a colleague is about to analyse a sample without proper centrifugation, I would pause the process, explain the importance of proper centrifugation, and ensure the sample is correctly processed. **In haematology**, if a staff member prepares a sample in the wrong anticoagulant tube, I would prevent the sample from being analysed incorrectly and guide them on using the correct tube.

After immediate correction, I would inform the senior or manager to ensure the incident is documented and the root cause is addressed, for example, by updating training or providing additional competency sessions. The aim is to turn the mistake into a learning opportunity without blaming the colleague, maintaining both quality standards and team morale.

Summary:

When a colleague makes a mistake, I ensure patient safety and laboratory quality are maintained by correcting the issue safely. I provide supportive guidance to the staff member to improve their practice and report the incident to a senior or manager for documentation and further review. For example, in biochemistry, I intervened when a sample was about to be analysed without centrifugation, and in haematology, I prevented analysis in the wrong tube type. This approach allows the colleague to learn, ensures standards are maintained, and helps prevent similar errors in the future.

Question 81:

Describe how you will lead a team.

Background:

Leadership within a pathology laboratory plays a crucial role in ensuring the smooth running of operations, compliance with ISO 15189 standards, and the delivery of accurate and timely results to support patient care. A good leader motivates and supports team members, encourages professional growth, and ensures quality and safety are never compromised. This question tests your understanding of effective leadership, delegation, communication, and accountability, which are vital to achieving laboratory objectives and maintaining a positive working culture.

Points to Consider:

- Understanding what effective leadership entails in a pathology laboratory.
- Ability to motivate, support, and guide team members.
- Leading by example and fostering teamwork.
- Awareness of the role of quality, communication, and continuous improvement.
- Practical examples to support your answer

Answer:

Leadership, to me, is about setting a clear vision, leading by example, and creating an environment where every team member feels valued and motivated to perform at their best. A good leader is approachable, organised, and ensures that quality and patient safety remain central to everything done in the laboratory.

For example, **in biochemistry**, when working as the lead on an out-of-hours shift, I prioritise tasks based on urgency such as processing emergency electrolytes or cardiac markers, while ensuring that my colleagues are confident and supported. I delegate roles clearly, ensure effective communication throughout the shift, and verify that all results are validated and reported accurately within turnaround times.

In haematology, I have led the team during high-workload periods, ensuring everyone remained calm and focused. I rotated staff between benches to balance workload, encouraged open communication when analyser issues arose, and liaised with senior staff or engineers for quick resolution. This approach not only improved efficiency but also strengthened team cohesion.

As a leader, I also prioritise training and development. When I notice a colleague struggling with a new analyser or process, I provide one-to-one support, go through the SOP together, and encourage reflective practice. I then escalate to the training officer or manager if further structured training is needed.

In microbiology, I once coordinated a small team responsible for urgent MRSA screening samples. By ensuring all positive results were communicated promptly to infection control, and by supporting less experienced staff with plate reading and interpretation, we maintained both accuracy and speed under pressure.

A key aspect of leadership is recognising and addressing mistakes constructively. I create a "no-blame" atmosphere, focusing on understanding the root cause and supporting colleagues through retraining or mentoring where needed as consistent with ISO 15189 and the laboratory's quality management system.

Lastly, I believe in continuous improvement. During a period of recurring instrument downtime, I organised a short debrief with the team to document the issue, identify possible causes, and implement a temporary manual backup plan. This proactive leadership minimised disruption and demonstrated accountability. I also, encourage and recommends staff for courses and trainings that would enhance understanding. Skills, and competencies.

Summary:

I believe leadership in the lab is about setting an example, maintaining quality, and empowering others. I lead by being approachable, communicating clearly, and supporting my team to work safely and efficiently. For example, in biochemistry, I've coordinated out-of-hours shifts where I delegated tasks, ensured critical samples were prioritised, and supported junior staff under pressure. My aim as a leader is always to create a supportive environment that promotes quality, learning, and patient safety while helping the team achieve its shared goals.

Question 82:

Tell us a scenario where you have worked as a team and where you have worked alone.

Background:

In the pathology laboratory, both teamwork and independent working are essential to maintaining service quality, accuracy, and timely patient care. Teamwork ensures efficiency during high workload or urgent situations, while working independently demonstrates competence, accountability, and confidence in handling laboratory processes safely. This question tests your understanding of how you adapt to both circumstances while maintaining ISO15189 and patient safety standards.

Points to Consider:

- The importance of teamwork in supporting quality and timely results.
- The need for independent work to demonstrate competence and accountability.
- How effective communication ensures smooth workflow in both cases.
- Emphasise patient safety, efficiency, and professionalism.
- Use practical examples to support your answer

Answer:

In the laboratory, there are times when teamwork is crucial to deliver timely and accurate results. For example, during staff shortages caused by annual or sick leave, or when there are technical downtimes involving analysers or the LIMS system. At other times, working alone is essential and it is expected that staff continue to demonstrate competence, confidence, and accountability while still maintaining patient safety. For example, during out-of-hours shifts.

Teamwork Example - Blood Transfusion (Routine & MHP)

In Blood Transfusion, teamwork and clear communication are essential, but accountability remains individual to maintain traceability and patient safety.

During routine work, different Biomedical Scientists perform different tasks. For example, one may receive and book samples, another centrifuge and load them, while others validate and issue units. However, during crossmatching, one scientist usually oversees the process from selecting blood and issuing compatible blood units to the patient. This support full traceability. However, a colleague can double-check the work to avoid oversight and that demonstrate teamwork in ensuring patient safety.

In contrast, during a Major Haemorrhage Protocol (MHP), the process becomes more urgent and require leading coordination. For example, I once received an MHP call for a trauma case. I verified patient identifiers over the phone on LIMS, prioritised the sample, selected and crossmatched suitable units, and issued them promptly. Meanwhile, my colleagues double-checked my crossmatch, assisted with blood packaging, and managed the documentation and delivery. This situation demonstrated how teamwork, communication, and role clarity under pressure directly impact patient outcomes.

Teamwork Example - Biochemistry

In Biochemistry, I once worked as part of a team during an analyser breakdown. We redistributed workload among several analysers and manually verified results for urgent samples such as electrolytes and cardiac enzymes. I communicated with the senior to prioritise urgent requests, while others liaised with wards and IT support. By working collaboratively, we minimised delays and ensured continuity of patient care despite the technical challenge.

Teamwork Example - Microbiology & Histopathology

In Microbiology, teamwork is essential, particularly during high-volume sample days. For example, during an outbreak screening, I collaborated with colleagues to log, plate, and incubate samples efficiently, ensuring accurate tracking in LIMS and timely reporting to infection control.

In Histopathology, teamwork is equally important during tissue embedding and sectioning. While one colleague prepares cassettes, another embeds, and another performs microtomy. This coordinated approach prevents backlogs and supports timely turnaround of critical biopsies.

Working Alone Example - Out-of-Hours / Haematology

Working alone is equally important, especially during out-of-hours shifts when Biomedical Scientists handle all urgent requests across departments. For example, during an OOH shift, I was responsible for Haematology and Biochemistry. A sample flagged as "possible blast cells" on the haematology analyser. I reviewed the smear microscopically, confirmed the abnormal cells, validated the result, and immediately phoned the finding to the on-call haematologist. Acting independently and confidently ensured prompt diagnosis and treatment for the patient.

These experiences have strengthened my ability to work effectively both independently and as part of a team, ensuring patient safety, communication, and having quality in mind.

Summary:

I understand that successful laboratory practice depends on balancing teamwork and independent working.

When working as part of a team, I prioritise clear communication, well-defined roles, and mutual support. For example, collaborating during a major haemorrhage in Blood Transfusion or managing analyser downtime in Biochemistry.

In the same vein, when working independently, such as during out-of-hours shifts, I rely on my competence, sound judgement, and adherence to SOPs to maintain service quality and ensure patient safety.

Both approaches complement each other - teamwork builds shared resilience and collaboration, while independent work

strengthens accountability and confidence. Together, they represent the core professional values expected of a Biomedical Scientist.

Question 83:

What CPDs are you doing now?

Background:

Continued professional development (CPD) is a requirement for Biomedical Scientists and other healthcare professionals to maintain their professional license, ensure competence, and enhance knowledge. CPD can take many forms, including academic study, research, conferences, training courses, and competency assessments. This question is testing your understanding of CPD's importance and your current engagement in professional development activities.

Points to consider:

- Demonstrate understanding of CPD and its role in maintaining professional standards and competence.
- Mention specific CPD activities undertaken in the past 12 months.
- Include different types of CPD: academic, research, conferences, training, and competency assessments.
- Provide practical examples of how these CPD activities improve knowledge and skills applicable in the lab.

Answer:

CPD is central to maintaining high professional standards and ensuring patient safety in laboratory practice. Over the past 12 months, I have actively engaged in several CPD activities across different formats:

- **Academic CPD:** I have undertaken a short course on molecular diagnostics, which has enhanced my understanding of PCR-based techniques and their application in infectious disease testing in the Microbiology department. This has allowed me to better interpret results and troubleshoot assays.

- **Research CPD:** I participated in a small departmental audit project evaluating pre-analytical sample handling in Biochemistry. This improved my understanding of how sample collection and handling can impact assay results and turnaround times.

- **Conference CPD:** I attended the UK Clinical Pathology Annual Conference, where I participated in workshops on laboratory automation and digital pathology. This provided insights into emerging technologies that could improve workflow efficiency and accuracy in Histopathology and Biochemistry.

- **Training CPD:** I completed internal competency updates for Haematology and Blood Transfusion procedures, including crossmatch verification and handling critical results. This ensures I remain confident and compliant with SOPs.

- **Competency assessments:** I regularly complete workplace-based competency assessments, including result validation in Biochemistry and specimen processing in Microbiology. These ensure that my practical skills remain up-to-date and consistent with ISO15189 standards.

Engaging in these CPD activities ensures that my knowledge and skills remain current, allows me to contribute effectively to patient care, and supports the department in maintaining high-quality standards.

Summary:

Currently, I am engaged in a range of CPD activities, including academic study in molecular diagnostics, research projects on pre-analytical handling, attending conferences on laboratory automation, internal training in Haematology and

Blood Transfusion, and regular competency assessments across departments. These activities ensure I remain competent, up to date with best practices, and able to contribute effectively to the team while maintaining patient safety and quality standards.

Question 84:

Tell us a scenario where you worked under pressure

Background:

Pathology laboratories are high-pressure environments where urgent patient needs, increased workload, staff shortages, or equipment downtime can create stress. How staff manage these situations without compromising patient safety or laboratory quality is critical. This question is testing your ability to remain calm, organised, and efficient while under pressure.

Points to consider:

- Demonstrate ability to remain calm under pressure
- Planning, prioritisation, and multitasking skills
- Ensuring patient safety and quality standards are maintained
- Provide practical examples to support your answer.

Answer:

Working under pressure is a common scenario in pathology laboratories. For example, **in a Biochemistry** department, there was an unexpected influx of samples due to an outbreak in a ward, combined with two staff members being off sick. I prioritised urgent samples, delegated tasks where possible, and ensured daily quality control checks were maintained. By focusing on planning, prioritising, and multitasking, we managed to process all critical samples within the expected turnaround time without compromising result accuracy.

In Blood Transfusion, I once managed a major haemorrhage alert while also processing routine samples. I quickly organised my workflow by taking responsibility for blood selection and crossmatching, while asking a colleague to double-check my preparation to prevent errors. At the same time, I coordinated communication with the ward to ensure prompt delivery of compatible units. Clear communication, effective role allocation, and strict adherence to SOPs enabled us to maintain patient safety even under significant time pressure.

In Microbiology, during a sudden increase in urgent sepsis samples, I had to process multiple cultures while ensuring proper documentation and immediate reporting of critical results. I used a systematic approach to prioritise high-risk samples first and maintained consistent checks against LIMS to avoid errors.

Summary:

I understand that working under pressure requires calmness, prioritisation, and efficient multitasking. Across departments like Biochemistry, Blood Transfusion, and Microbiology, I ensure patient safety, adhere to SOPs, and communicate effectively with colleagues and wards. These experiences have strengthened my ability to deliver accurate results promptly even in high-pressure situations.

Question 85:

Tell us a scenario where you have had to prioritise your work.

Background:

Pathology laboratories are often busy environments with multiple samples, tests, and urgent requests arriving simultaneously. Prioritisation is essential to ensure that critical results are processed quickly, while maintaining accuracy and safety. This question is testing your understanding of how to organise tasks, manage competing demands, and apply professional judgement to maintain patient care and laboratory quality.

Points to consider:

- Understanding urgency and criticality of different samples (e.g., A&E, ITU, urgent biochemistry panels, histopathology biopsies).
- Using SOPs and Trust guidelines to prioritise workflow.
- Balancing routine workload with urgent tasks.
- Use practical example to support your answer.

Answer:

In a busy pathology laboratory, prioritisation is key to maintaining patient safety and service quality. For example, **in Biochemistry,** I once had multiple samples to process, including routine outpatient samples and an urgent potassium and troponin profile from A&E for a patient with suspected myocardial infarction. I immediately prioritised the urgent A&E sample, processed it, and phoned the result to the ward, while ensuring routine samples were queued according to standard TAT.

Similarly, **in Haematology**, I had a scenario where a patient's full blood count required urgent review for suspected sepsis, while routine outpatient samples were waiting. I prioritised the urgent sample, validated the results, and communicated with the clinical team, before completing routine testing.

In Blood Transfusion, prioritisation is vital during urgent requests, such as for a patient needing crossmatched blood. I ensured the patient's sample was processed immediately, selected compatible units, performed necessary checks, crossmatched the patient sample (plasma) against the donor red cell, and issued the compactible blood while other routine transfusion samples waited.

Even **in Histopathology and Microbiology,** prioritisation is required. For instance, if a tissue biopsy needs urgent reporting due to suspected malignancy, or a microbiology sample indicates potential sepsis, these tasks are prioritised over routine non-urgent specimens.

By applying these principles, I ensure that urgent tasks are completed on time, while routine work continues within its expected TAT, so patient care is maintained, and no tasks are neglected.

Summary:

In my experience, prioritisation involves assessing urgency, understanding the clinical context, and applying laboratory SOPs to manage multiple tasks efficiently. For example, I prioritised urgent A&E samples in Biochemistry, rapid blood requests in Transfusion, and critical tissue biopsies in Histopathology, while ensuring routine work continued appropriately. This approach safeguards patient safety, maintains quality standards, and demonstrates the effective time management and decision-making skills essential for a Biomedical Scientist.

Question 86:

Tell us where you were working that you encountered a problem and how did you solve it.

Background:

In the pathology laboratory, unexpected challenges can occur at any time ranging from equipment failure to communication breakdowns or sample quality issues. How we respond to these problems reflects our professionalism, problem-solving ability, and understanding of quality and patient safety. This question tests your ability to stay calm, follow SOPs, and resolve problems efficiently without compromising laboratory standards.

Points to consider:

- Identify and describe the problem clearly.
- Show your investigative and problem-solving approach.
- Explain the steps taken to correct and prevent recurrence
- Demonstrate teamwork, communication, and adherence to SOPs.
- Use examples to support your answer.

Answer:

In Biochemistry, I once encountered a problem where the main analyser failed calibration in the middle of a busy shift. I immediately stopped processing new samples, checked maintenance records, and performed basic troubleshooting according to the SOP - cleaning probes and re-running calibrators. When the issue persisted, I escalated to the senior biomedical scientist and contacted the engineering support team. To prevent delay in patient results, I identified urgent samples such as A&E and ITU cases and arranged for them to be processed on a backup analyser. Once the problem was resolved, I verified QC performance before resuming routine testing. This approach ensured continuity of service and patient safety.

In Haematology, I encountered an incident where an analyser flagged abnormal white cell scattergrams for multiple samples. I reviewed the flags and examined a peripheral blood film manually, confirming the presence of blasts in one patient. I immediately informed the senior BMS, who contacted the consultant haematologist. This early identification contributed to the urgent diagnosis of acute leukaemia. The experience highlighted the importance of combining analyser data with manual verification and teamwork in supporting clinical decision-making.

In Blood Transfusion, a problem arose when a patient sample arrived with mismatched identifiers between the tube and request form. According to SOP, I did not process the sample but informed the ward immediately to recollect and correctly label it. I documented the incident in the non-conformance log. The situation reinforced the importance of strict adherence to sample identification policies to prevent potential transfusion errors.

In Histopathology, I encountered a case where tissue cassettes were mislabelled due to a printing error. I stopped the embedding process, segregated affected samples, and informed the senior BMS and pathologist. After reviewing the block log and request forms, we confirmed the correct identities and re-labelled them correctly before embedding. The issue was later raised in the quality meeting, and a double-check step was introduced for cassette printing to prevent recurrence.

Finally, **in Microbiology,** I once noticed that the incubator temperature was fluctuating beyond the acceptable range. I recorded the deviation, informed the senior, and transferred the plates to a functioning incubator. I also checked recently incubated cultures to ensure no growth issues occurred. Engineering later replaced the thermostat. My quick response prevented any compromise in result reliability.

Summary:

I have faced different challenges such as analyser breakdowns, sample identification issues, and equipment faults. My approach is always consistent: stay calm, investigate systematically, follow SOPs, communicate with seniors, and document actions. These experiences have strengthened my problem-solving skills, improved my attention to detail, and reinforced my commitment to patient safety and quality laboratory practice.

Question 87:

What mistake have you made since you started working, and how did you solve it?

Background:

Mistakes are part of every learning process, especially in a complex and high-pressure environment like the pathology laboratory. What truly defines professionalism is the ability to recognise, correct, and learn from these mistakes in line with ISO15189, HCPC standards, and the laboratory's quality management system (QMS). This question assesses your integrity, reflection, and commitment to patient safety and continuous improvement.

Points to consider:

- Mistakes can occur at any stage - pre-analytical, analytical, or post-analytical.
- Importance of identifying and correcting errors quickly.
- Reporting mistakes through appropriate channels to maintain transparency.
- Learning from experience and preventing recurrence.
- Reflecting honesty, accountability, and growth.
- Use practical examples to support your answer.

Answer:

I believe that acknowledging and learning from mistakes is an essential part of professional growth and maintaining a strong quality culture in the laboratory.

For example, during my early days **in Biochemistry,** I validated a patient's electrolytes result that seemed inconsistent with their previous history. On review, I noticed that the sample was haemolysed, which had caused a falsely elevated potassium result. I immediately contacted the ward to request a repeat sample, re-analysed the new sample, and corrected the report. The incident was documented in the non-conformance log, which allowed the team to discuss ways to improve sample quality checks at pre-analysis.

In Haematology, I once reviewed a blood film that didn't correlate with the automated differential count. Upon reflection, I realised that the wrong slide had been selected from the batch. I quickly repeated the smear, verified the correct findings, and reported the issue to the senior. The incident was later used as a discussion point during our team meeting to reinforce the importance of proper labelling and slide handling.

In Blood Transfusion, I once selected a blood unit for issue but noticed that the barcode scanner had failed. Before issuing, I double-checked the unit details manually and realised that the blood group didn't match the patient record. I stopped the issue, quarantined the unit, and informed the senior biomedical scientist.

The event emphasised the importance of not bypassing manual verification even when technology fails.

In Microbiology, there was an instance where a culture plate was mislabelled during processing, which could have led to an incorrect report. I identified the error when colony morphology did not match the expected organism from the clinical notes. I immediately informed the senior, repeated the culture using the original sample, and documented the incident. This taught me the importance of cross-checking patient identifiers and clinical details during every processing stage.

Similarly, **in Histopathology,** I once encountered a mix-up between cassettes during embedding due to a distraction at the workstation. I recognised the error when the tissue description didn't match the request form, immediately stopped the process, segregated the samples, and alerted the senior BMS. The case was resolved through joint review, and I later contributed to developing a new double-check procedure before embedding.

Summary:

I understand that mistakes can happen, but how we respond to them reflects our professionalism and commitment to patient safety. Whenever I have made an error, I take responsibility, act promptly to correct it, and report it through the appropriate channels. I also reflect on what went wrong, review the relevant SOPs, and share my experience with colleagues to help prevent recurrence.

These experiences across Biochemistry, Haematology, Blood Transfusion, Microbiology, and Histopathology have taught me to remain vigilant, uphold quality standards, and never become complacent. Each mistake I have encountered has strengthened my competence, improved my attention to detail, and deepened my understanding of the importance of teamwork, communication, and continuous improvement in delivering safe and reliable patient care.

Question 88:

Tell us where u have a suggested to improve a lab, what is the suggestion and how it improved the Lab quality.

Background:

Continuous improvement is at the heart of every quality-driven laboratory. ISO15189 emphasises that all staff, regardless of role or grade, should be encouraged to identify areas for improvement and contribute to service development. This question is testing your ability to recognise inefficiencies, suggest practical solutions, and understand how improvements align with patient safety, turnaround times (TAT), and overall laboratory quality.

Points to consider:

- The importance of staff involvement in service improvement.
- Example of a specific improvement suggestion made.
- The impact of the suggestion on quality, efficiency, or patient outcomes.
- Reflection on teamwork and QMS principles (corrective and preventive actions).
- Use of practical examples to support the answer.

Answer:

I believe that continuous improvement is everyone's responsibility, not just the managers. I always take note of areas where small changes can make a big difference to workflow, efficiency, or quality.

For example, while working in **Biochemistry**, I observed that urgent samples from the emergency department were sometimes delayed because they became mixed with routine specimens at reception. Recognising the potential impact on patient care, I suggested introducing a clearly labelled "urgent samples" tray positioned in a separate, dedicated area. This simple change allowed reception staff to identify and prioritise urgent requests more easily, ensuring they were loaded and processed without delay. The idea was discussed at a team meeting, approved by the senior BMS, and implemented successfully. As a result, turnaround times for urgent samples improved noticeably, and feedback from clinical staff was overwhelmingly positive.

In Haematology, I once suggested creating a daily analyser maintenance checklist to be signed by the staff on duty. Before this, some maintenance steps were occasionally missed during busy shifts. My suggestion ensured accountability and consistency, which led to fewer instrument errors and smoother operation.

In Blood Transfusion, I noticed that staff often had to search through several folders to find updated manufacturer inserts for reagents and consumables. I proposed creating a centralised digital folder on Q-Pulse with all current inserts uploaded and regularly updated. This reduced confusion, saved time, and ensured we always worked with up-to-date manufacturer information supporting compliance with ISO15189 documentation requirements.

In Microbiology, during a review of culture worklists, I observed that some repeat samples were being processed unnecessarily before the first set of results were finalised. I suggested adding a simple flagging system in LIMS to alert staff when a repeat specimen was already in process. This reduced duplication, reagent use, and workload, improving efficiency.

Similarly, **in Histopathology,** I proposed using a colour-coded tray system for specimens at different stages of processing (e.g., embedding, microtomy, staining). This made it easier to track workflow and reduced the risk of mix-ups or delays, especially during peak workloads.

Summary:

I believe improvement suggestions, no matter how small, can have a meaningful impact on laboratory performance. By observing workflow issues and thinking proactively, I have been able to contribute to better turnaround times, improved traceability, and enhanced staff efficiency.

In each case, I ensured that my suggestions were raised through the proper channels, discussed with seniors or managers, and supported by QMS principles. These experiences have taught me that improvement is an ongoing process driven by teamwork, good communication, and a shared commitment to patient safety and service excellence.

Question 89:

Tell us where you have suggested to improve a lab, what is the suggestion, and how could it have improved the lab if it was implemented.

Background:

Continuous improvement is one of the cornerstones of ISO15189 and an essential element of a laboratory's Quality Management System (QMS). Biomedical Scientists are expected not only to carry out analytical tasks but also to identify potential areas of improvement that enhance efficiency, accuracy, and safety. This question assesses your ability to recognise process gaps, propose practical solutions, and understand the potential impact of your suggestions.

Points to consider:

- Importance of continuous improvement within ISO15189 framework.
- Examples of practical suggestions made to improve workflow or quality.
- Explain how your suggestion added value (e.g., efficiency, quality, turnaround time, safety).
- Reflect on how it could have further improved laboratory operations if fully implemented.

Answer:

Continuous improvement is a vital aspect of laboratory practice, ensuring that processes evolve to meet clinical demands, reduce errors, and support ISO15189 standards. In my previous role, I identified several areas where workflow and efficiency could be improved through staff-led initiatives.

For example, **in Haematology,** I noticed delays in sample processing during peak times because all urgent samples were being sent directly to one analyser. I suggested implementing a triage system where one analyser was designated for urgent work and another for routine samples. **If implemented,** this would have improved turnaround time for emergency samples such as those from A&E, ensuring that urgent results were available more quickly for clinical decision-making.

In Biochemistry, I suggested introducing a visual "Pending Results Board" within the LIMS interface to highlight incomplete or delayed samples. This would have enabled biomedical scientist's response and support staff to identify sample pending early, reducing turnaround time breaches and preventing unnecessary repeat requests from clinicians.

In Microbiology, I proposed standardising communication with the clinical team by creating a daily update sheet for significant isolates (such as MRSA or ESBL). **If implemented,** this would have strengthened collaboration between the laboratory and infection control, ensuring timely clinical intervention.

Similarly, during my experience **in Histopathology**, I recommended adding an internal log to track specimen fixation time before processing. This would have helped maintain tissue integrity and reduced the need for repeat embedding, ultimately improving diagnostic quality.

Each of these suggestions focused on improving efficiency, communication, and compliance with quality standards. Some were adopted immediately, while others were discussed for potential implementation during service improvement meetings.

Summary:

I believe laboratory improvement is a continuous process driven by observation, collaboration, and feedback. Whether it involves improving turnaround times, communication channels, or workflow efficiency, my suggestions have always been aimed at maintaining high-quality patient results and ensuring ISO15189 compliance. Even when suggestions are not fully implemented, the process itself fosters a culture of innovation and accountability, which is essential qualities for a Biomedical Scientist.

Question 90:

What do you understand by going the extra mile in the laboratory?

Background:

"Going the extra mile" in the laboratory means doing more than what is normally expected to ensure quality patient care, efficiency, and safety. It reflects a proactive attitude, teamwork, and commitment to improving laboratory services. Biomedical Scientists and other laboratory professionals are often faced with situations that require extra effort to maintain service delivery, meet turnaround times, and support patient outcomes, even under pressure. This question tests your motivation, dedication, and sense of responsibility toward patient care and service excellence.

Points to consider:

- What "going the extra mile" means in laboratory practice.
- The importance of putting patients first.
- Examples of going beyond normal duties to ensure service continuity or improvement.
- How it links to teamwork, professionalism, and Trust values.

Answer:

For me, going the extra mile in the laboratory means going beyond minimum requirements to uphold quality, safety, and trust. It reflects a commitment not only to my professional role, but also to the patients whose care depends on accurate and timely results.

One such moment occurred in Blood Transfusion during a particularly busy on-call night. Although my shift had officially ended, I stayed on to support a colleague handling an urgent massive haemorrhage protocol case. Recognising the critical nature of the situation, I assisted in preparing emergency O negative units and carefully double-checking the crossmatched blood to ensure accuracy. By doing so, we avoided unnecessary delays and helped support the clinical team as they worked to stabilise a severely bleeding patient.

In Biochemistry, I once noticed that an analyser showed inconsistent quality control (QC) results close to the end of the shift. Instead of leaving it for the next team, I stayed a bit longer to repeat the QC, run calibrations, and document the findings. This prevented reporting potentially incorrect patient results and avoided unnecessary panic for the clinicians.

Similarly, **in Microbiology,** when a critical blood culture result indicated a possible Gram-negative sepsis, I immediately phoned the ward even though it was slightly outside my assigned area. This ensured prompt treatment and likely prevented deterioration in the patient's condition.

In Histopathology, I supported the biomedical support workers to prioritise urgent biopsies for same-day processing, ensuring that cancer diagnostic cases were not delayed.

These actions, although not mandatory, reflect going the extra mile by doing what is necessary to protect patients and support colleagues. It also shows commitment to maintaining high laboratory standards as required by ISO15180 and Trust policies.

Summary:

Going the extra mile in the laboratory means putting patient care, quality, and teamwork above convenience. It involves small but important actions like staying late to complete urgent work, supporting colleagues under pressure, or identifying and resolving issues before they escalate. These extra efforts promote efficiency, strengthen team spirit, and ultimately contribute to better patient outcomes.

Question 91:

Tell me about yourself

Background:

This is one of the most common opening questions in an interview. It allows you to introduce yourself professionally and show how your background, experience, and passion align with the role of a Biomedical Scientist. The aim is to demonstrate your understanding of the position, your enthusiasm for laboratory science, and the unique value you bring to the team.

Points to consider:

- Mention your passion for science and patient care.
- Briefly outline your academic and professional background.
- Highlight relevant experience and competencies gained in the laboratory or healthcare environment.
- Demonstrate key skills (e.g., teamwork, communication, attention to detail, problem-solving).
- Link your values and approach to the Trust or organisational values.
- Use practical examples to support your points.

Answer:

Thank you for the opportunity to introduce myself. My name is [Your Name], and I am a Biomedical Scientist with a strong passion for delivering high-quality laboratory services that directly support patient diagnosis and treatment.

I began my journey in healthcare as a [for example: medical laboratory assistant / healthcare assistant / phlebotomist], where I developed a deep appreciation for how every part of the laboratory process contributes to patient care. That early experience taught me the importance of teamwork, communication, and accuracy in a healthcare setting.

Academically, I hold a degree in Biomedical Science and am HCPC-registered. During my training and work placements, I gained experience across several key laboratory disciplines, including Haematology, Blood Transfusion, Biochemistry, and Microbiology. Each department offered a different perspective on how laboratory science underpins patient care. In Haematology, I became confident in operating automated analysers such as the Sysmex XN line and interpreting abnormal results, while in Blood Transfusion I developed practical expertise in antibody screening, crossmatching, and the safe issue of blood components in line with established standards and procedures.

Beyond routine duties, I have also sought opportunities to contribute to service improvement. In Biochemistry, for instance, I proposed the introduction of a simple daily bench quality-control checklist to monitor equipment readiness and reduce analyser downtime. Although small, this change helped streamline workflow, improve turnaround times, and reinforced the value of proactive quality management in the laboratory.

I consider myself a collaborative and adaptable professional and I enjoy working as part of a team but can also work independently when required, especially during out-of-hours shifts where efficiency and decision-making are key. I always strive to maintain the highest standards of laboratory practice and patient safety.

Looking ahead, I am passionate about continuous learning and development. I am actively involved in CPD activities such as attending webinars, reviewing EQA outcomes, and mentoring junior staff to build confidence and competence. I believe that growth through shared learning helps improve both individual performance and the overall quality of laboratory services.

Summary:

I am a dedicated Biomedical Scientist with a strong academic foundation, hands-on laboratory experience, and a genuine passion for improving patient care through quality laboratory practice. My diverse experience from Haematology and Transfusion to Biochemistry and Microbiology has shaped me into a well-rounded professional who values teamwork, precision, and continuous improvement. I am eager to contribute these qualities to your team and continue to develop within your department.

Question 92:

How do you get out of a difficult situation?

Background:

In the laboratory, challenges can arise unexpectedly such as equipment malfunction, unclear results, or time-sensitive situations that require urgent decision-making. Biomedical Scientists must be able to handle such situations calmly and professionally, maintaining compliance with laboratory SOPs, ISO15189 standards, and professional codes of conduct (such as HCPC). The key is recognising personal and professional limits, asking for help when appropriate, and using established laboratory structures to resolve the issue without compromising patient safety or result accuracy.

Points to consider:

- Recognising when a situation is beyond your competence or authority.
- Consulting colleagues, seniors, or managers for guidance.
- Referring to SOPs, manufacturer manuals, or regulatory guidelines (e.g., UKAS, MHRA, BSH, HTA).

- Maintaining accurate documentation of the incident and corrective actions.
- Using the experience as a learning opportunity for improvement.
- Use practical examples to support your points.

Answer:

In the laboratory, I believe that recognising when to ask for help is an important part of professionalism. If I encounter a difficult situation, my first step is always to remain calm, assess the issue, and determine whether it's something I can resolve safely within my scope of practice.

Whenever I encounter uncertainty in the laboratory, I return to the procedures and guidance that underpin our work. Knowing when to pause, check, and seek support is as important as technical skill. If a situation falls outside my experience, I escalate it to a senior colleague, recognising that patient safety must always come first.

I remember one occasion in Blood Transfusion when a patient's antibody screen produced a positive result that did not fit any familiar pattern. Rather than forcing a conclusion, I stopped the process and reviewed the guidance before discussing the case with a senior biomedical scientist. We examined the results together and agreed that the safest option was to send the sample to a specialist reference laboratory for further investigation. That decision ensured the patient received appropriate and safe transfusion support, and it reinforced for me the value of professional humility and teamwork in laboratory practice.

In another scenario **in Biochemistry**, we once had an analyser give inconsistent QC results just before the morning workload. I immediately ran a repeat QC, checked reagent expiry date, and reviewed the calibration log. When the problem persisted, I escalated it to the duty senior and recorded it as a non-conformance on Q-Pulse. The senior liaised with the service engineer, and we temporarily switched testing to the backup analyser. This ensured service continuity while maintaining quality assurance.

Similarly, **in Microbiology,** if I have difficulty identifying an organism. For example, when biochemical test results are inconclusive, I would consult the UK Standards for Microbiology Investigations (UK SMI) or discuss it with a senior or consultant microbiologist before releasing any result.

Overall, I never hesitate to ask questions or seek help from colleagues, seniors, or managers if I am unsure. The key is to communicate effectively and escalate appropriately while documenting all actions taken. This approach aligns with the UKAS ISO15189, HCPC professional standards and ensures the patient's safety is never compromised.

Summary:

In summary, my approach to difficult situations is guided by professionalism, teamwork, and adherence to established laboratory standards. I stay calm, assess the situation, and use available resources such as SOPs, MHRA, BSH, and UKAS guidelines. When unsure, I seek help from senior colleagues or managers, ensuring that all actions are documented. For example, consulting a senior during complex antibody identification in Blood Transfusion or escalating analyser failures in Biochemistry ensures timely and accurate resolution. Through this approach, I not only protect patient safety but also build confidence and competence by learning from experienced colleagues. Difficult situations, when handled correctly, become opportunities for professional growth and quality improvement.

Question 93:

As we are upgrading from one supplier to another, what do you suggest we do in setting it up?

Background:

When a laboratory upgrades from one supplier to another, whether it is for reagents, analysers, or software systems. it is usually not just a simple swap. Each change must go through a structured verification, validation, and change control process to ensure the new system performs to the manufacturer's specification and meets ISO15189 quality standards. This process ensures that analytical performance, accuracy, and reproducibility are maintained, and that patient results remain consistent and reliable during and after the transition.

Points to consider:

- Change control and risk assessment process.
- Verification and validation in line with ISO15189.
- Communication with manufacturer/supplier and multidisciplinary team.
- Comparison studies with existing systems.
- Staff training, competency assessment, and SOP review.
- Quality assurance measures (IQC, EQA, and measurement of uncertainty).
- Documentation and UKAS evidence of traceability.
- Use practical examples to support your points.

Answer:

Upgrading from one supplier to another is a significant process that must be handled systematically to maintain quality and ensure patient safety. My first step would be to initiate a change control procedure in line with the laboratory's quality management system (QMS) and ISO15189 requirements.

The process begins with a careful risk assessment, identifying potential issues such as analytical variation, reagent compatibility, or differences in data interfaces. This assessment is reviewed by the senior team or quality lead before any changes are introduced.

Once approved, the supplier is required to provide full installation, operational, and performance qualification documentation. Following installation, the laboratory team carries out verification and validation testing to ensure that the new equipment or reagents perform as expected and are consistent with the system they replace. These steps help ensure that any change is introduced safely, thoughtfully, and without compromising the reliability of patient results.

For example, **in Biochemistry,** if we are upgrading from Roche to Abbott analysers, I would conduct parallel testing of running patient and quality control samples on both systems and comparing results statistically (e.g., regression analysis, bias, precision). The verification would include testing at normal, high, and low ranges to ensure linearity and accuracy.

In Haematology, if switching from Sysmex to Beckman Coulter analysers, similar comparison and correlation studies should be performed for parameters like Hb, WBC, platelets, and differential counts. Abnormal samples should also be included to confirm the analyser's ability to flag pathology correctly.

For **Blood Transfusion,** if switching reagent suppliers for antibody screening or crossmatch testing, it is crucial to validate the new reagent batches using known positive and negative samples and ensure the results match reference methods. In addition, staff should be trained on any procedural differences, and SOPs updated accordingly.

Throughout this process, internal quality control (IQC) and external quality assessment (EQA) must be re-established and reviewed to confirm continued compliance. Additionally, measurement of uncertainty (MU) should be recalculated to ensure analytical reliability.

Finally, all staff involved must receive training and competency assessment on the new system before it goes live. All documentation - including validation reports, risk assessments, training records, and updated SOPs should be stored on Q-Pulse or equivalent system for UKAS audit evidence.

Summary:

Upgrading from one supplier to another requires a structured and documented approach that includes risk assessment, validation, verification, and training. The process must follow ISO15189 and UKAS standards to ensure analytical accuracy and patient safety are maintained. For example, performing parallel testing between Roche and Abbott analysers in Biochemistry, or validating new antibody screening reagents in Blood Transfusion, ensures continuity of quality and confidence in results. Through proper documentation, comparison studies, and competency training, the laboratory can transition smoothly without compromising service quality or patient outcomes.

Question 94:

Give us a challenging situation you have faced and how you overcame it.

Background:

Working in a pathology laboratory can sometimes present challenging situations whether due to high workload, equipment failure, unexpected analytical errors, or staffing shortages. What matters most however, is not just identifying the challenge, but demonstrating critical thinking, professionalism, and collaboration to resolve the issue without compromising patient safety or turnaround times (TAT). This question tests your resilience, teamwork, and ability to stay calm and solution-focused in difficult situations.

Points to Consider:

- Identify a realistic and relevant challenge you have experienced in the lab.
- Describe how you handled it calmly and professionally.
- Show your problem-solving process - what steps you took to resolve it.

- Emphasise communication, teamwork, and adherence to SOP and quality standards.
- Highlight what you learned from the experience.
- Use practical examples across different departments.

Answer:

One challenging situation I faced occurred **in Biochemistry,** when our main analyser suddenly went down during a busy weekend shift, just as we received a large batch of urgent A&E and ITU samples. This situation could easily have caused significant delay in TAT and affected patient care.

I immediately followed the analyser downtime SOP by first confirming the error code and performing the basic troubleshooting steps such as checking reagent levels, recalibrating, and restarting the system. When the problem persisted, I escalated it to the senior on-call Biomedical Scientist and the engineer support line while maintaining communication with the clinical areas, informing them about potential delays.

To maintain service, I prioritised urgent samples and transferred them to the back-up analyser after performing verification and QC checks to ensure result reliability. I also contacted the nearby hospital within the Trust to arrange a contingency plan in case the backup failed.

This experience taught me the importance of staying calm under pressure, communicating effectively, and adhering to established contingency protocols.

Similarly, **in Blood Transfusion**, a challenging situation occurred when there was a major haemorrhage call during a night shift while the ward was still sending group and screen samples. I had to act quickly verified the sample on LIMS, selected suitable emergency O-negative units, and ensured that group-specific blood was crossmatched and issued promptly once results became available. A colleague helped double-check all compatibility paperwork, and we communicated clearly with the clinical team throughout.

The situation reinforced the value of teamwork and vigilance during high-pressure scenarios.

In Microbiology, I once faced a challenge when a contamination issue was suspected in urine culture plates due to a batch of faulty loops. I reported the incident through the non-conformance system, participated in the root cause investigation, and helped review the SOP to prevent future recurrence.

Each of these experiences has improved my ability to manage stress, prioritise tasks, and make decisions confidently while maintaining quality and patient safety.

Summary:

Challenges are inevitable in the laboratory, but how we respond defines our professionalism. I handle challenges by staying calm, following SOPs, communicating effectively, and seeking support when necessary. For example, when our biochemistry analyser failed, I ensured continuity of service through troubleshooting, prioritisation, and teamwork without compromising patient care. These experiences have strengthened my resilience, confidence, and understanding of how collaboration and adherence to quality systems can turn a difficult situation into a learning opportunity.

Question 95:

Your colleague you are supposed to hand over to did not come early for the shift, what will you do?

Background:

Pathology laboratories operate as essential, round-the-clock services, where effective handover between shifts is vital to maintaining continuity of patient care. When a colleague due to take over a shift is delayed, it can disrupt workflow, delay the reporting of results, and place pressure on the service if not managed appropriately. Situations like this highlight the importance of professional accountability, clear communication, and a shared understanding of handover responsibilities within the laboratory.

Points to consider:

- Importance of a proper handover for patient safety and service continuity.
- Following Trust policy and escalation procedure when a colleague is late.
- Avoid leaving the bench unattended by staying until safe cover is provided.
- Communicate effectively with seniors, shift coordinator, or duty manager.
- Maintain professionalism by not making assumptions or express frustration.
- Use practical example to support your answer.

Answer:

If my colleague who is meant to take over the shift does not arrive on time, my first priority would be to ensure continuity of service and patient safety. I would remain on duty until appropriate cover is available by ensuring that no urgent samples, transfusions, or analyser processes are left unattended.

For example, **in Blood Transfusion**, if I am on a night shift and my relief is delayed, I would continue to monitor any ongoing crossmatches, verify urgent results, and remain available in case of an emergency call such as a massive haemorrhage protocol. I would never leave the laboratory unattended, as doing so could pose a significant risk to patient safety.

I would contact the colleague to confirm expected arrival time. Also, I would make the senior Biomedical Scientist, shift coordinator, or on-call manager aware of the situation. This allows them to further contact the colleague, confirm their estimated arrival time, or arrange for temporary cover if necessary.

Similarly, **in Biochemistry or Haematology,** if I am about to finish a busy shift and the next shift scientist is running late, I would continue to monitor analyser status, review pending results, and ensure QC is within range so that the service continues smoothly when the next staff arrives. I would document any critical information in the handover log or LIMS handover notes to maintain traceability.

If the colleague arrives later, I will provide a clear and concise handover, explaining any pending work, issues, or urgent samples. I would avoid showing frustration, as professionalism and teamwork are essential in maintaining a supportive working environment.

Practical Example:

I recall one weekend shift in Haematology when the colleague due to relieve me was delayed by unexpected transport problems. I informed the senior biomedical scientist and remained on duty for an additional forty-five minutes to ensure that urgent samples from ITU and A&E were completed without delay. When my colleague arrived, I carried out a thorough handover, including analyser logs, quality control performance, and any outstanding work. Later, the senior thanked me for helping to maintain continuity of service, and the incident was noted in the shift record as an example of good professional conduct.

That said, if lateness were to become a repeated issue without a genuine reason, it would need to be addressed more formally. Persistent delays can disrupt workflow, place unnecessary pressure on colleagues, and risk turnaround times for patient results. Escalating such concerns to the senior team allows them to be managed fairly and constructively, while also ensuring that any underlying personal or work-related issues are identified and appropriately supported.

Summary:

In such situations, my approach would always prioritise patient safety, service continuity, and professionalism. I would remain on duty until cover arrives, inform the senior or duty manager, and document all actions taken. Even though it can be inconvenient, maintaining laboratory service is the most important priority. By handling the situation calmly and

responsibly, I help uphold the standards of ISO15189, protect patient care, and demonstrate teamwork and reliability, which is one of the key qualities for any Biomedical Scientist.

Question 96:

What IT skills do you have that are relevant to this post?

Background:

Information technology plays a vital role in modern pathology laboratories. It supports data entry, analysis, traceability, communication, and compliance with ISO15189 standards. Biomedical Scientists must be competent in using various IT systems, including Laboratory Information Management Systems (LIMS), analyser interfaces, middleware, and quality management software. This question tests your ability to use IT effectively and your understanding of how digital tools contribute to laboratory efficiency, accuracy, and quality assurance.

Points to consider:

- Importance of IT in laboratory workflow and quality assurance
- Examples of IT systems used (LIMS, Q-Pulse, middleware, EQA portals, data analysis tools)
- How IT improves patient safety and turnaround times
- Data security and confidentiality (GDPR awareness)
- Use examples to support your answer.

Answer:

IT skills are an essential part of my daily work as a Biomedical Scientist. I regularly use a range of laboratory and administrative systems that support analytical accuracy, quality management, and traceability.

For example, **in Haematology and Biochemistry,** I use LIMS (Telepath, LabCentre, MediTech, Cerna, Bank Manager, WinPath) to register, track, and authorise patient samples, ensuring that all patient information is correctly entered and results are traceable from receipt to release. I also work with middleware systems such as Instrument Manager or LabCentre, which link analysers to LIMS, allowing automatic result verification and flagging of abnormal results for review.

In Blood Transfusion, I use electronic blood tracking systems and BBL (Blood Bank LIMS modules) to crossmatch, issue, and document blood units. I am familiar with using barcode scanners and handheld devices for patient verification to comply with MHRA and UKAS requirements on traceability.

In Microbiology, I have experience using digital platforms such as Telepath or WinPath, which help track culture progress, enter sensitivity results, and link to antimicrobial stewardship reports. Similarly, **in Histopathology,** I have used digital pathology systems and image databases for slide tracking and result reporting.

In addition, I use Q-Pulse for document control, incident reporting (or DATIX for incident reporting), and managing quality records. I also have experience with EQA portals for submitting results and downloading performance reports. For data handling, I am proficient in Microsoft Excel and Word, which I use to record QC data, generate trend charts, and prepare audit summaries.

I understand the importance of data protection and confidentiality, adhering to GDPR principles, and ensuring that patient information is securely handled at all times.

Summary:

My IT skills cover the full spectrum of laboratory operations, from sample processing and data analysis to quality management and reporting. I am confident in using LIMS, middleware, Q-Pulse, and Microsoft Office applications to maintain efficiency, traceability, and compliance with ISO15189 standards. These skills allow mo to work accurately, adapt quickly to new technologies, and support continuous improvement in laboratory practice.

Question 97:

What do you understand about UKAS and MHRA, and how do they relate to laboratory practice? OR

Explain the roles and differences between UKAS and MHRA in the pathology laboratory.

Background:

Pathology laboratories in the UK must operate under strict regulatory and accreditation frameworks to ensure quality, safety, and reliability of patient results. Two of the key bodies responsible for maintaining these standards are UKAS (United Kingdom Accreditation Service) and MHRA (Medicines and Healthcare products Regulatory Agency). Understanding their roles helps Biomedical Scientists maintain compliance, uphold quality standards, and support patient safety.

Points to consider:

- What UKAS and MHRA stand for
- Their main responsibilities and scope in pathology laboratories
- Differences between the two
- How they work together to maintain quality and compliance
- Practical examples (inspection, documentation, traceability, and non-conformance management)

Answer:

Both UKAS and MHRA play vital roles in maintaining high-quality and safe laboratory services, but they focus on slightly different areas of regulation and accreditation.

In the UK, the United Kingdom Accreditation Service (UKAS) is responsible for assessing and accrediting pathology laboratories against ISO 15189 standards. Its role is to ensure that laboratories are technically competent, use properly validated methods, adhere to standard operating procedures, and operate within robust quality management systems.

During UKAS inspections, assessors examine a wide range of laboratory practices, including sample traceability, quality control records, staff training, document control systems, and internal audit processes. When a non-conformance is identified, such as incomplete documentation or a deviation from an established procedure, the laboratory is required to record the issue and implement corrective and preventive actions within an agreed timeframe. These processes are central to maintaining consistency, accountability, and trust in laboratory services.

MHRA (Medicines and Healthcare products Regulatory Agency), on the other hand, regulates blood transfusion services, medical devices, and medicines. In pathology, MHRA is particularly relevant to Blood Transfusion Laboratories, ensuring compliance with the Blood Safety and Quality Regulations (BSQR 2005).

The MHRA focuses on areas such as traceability of blood and blood components, cold chain monitoring, equipment calibration, incident reporting through SABRE (Serious Adverse Blood Reaction and Events), and ensuring staff training and competency. For example, during MHRA inspections, assessors may trace a blood unit from issue to transfusion and review documentation to confirm full traceability and temperature compliance.

While UKAS ensures that the laboratory meets quality and technical standards, MHRA ensures that all blood and blood components used in patient care are safe, traceable, and comply with legal regulations.

In practice, both agencies complement each other (Table 1). For example, in Blood Transfusion, UKAS assesses the lab's QMS under ISO15189, while MHRA ensures regulatory compliance under BSQR. A finding from either inspection can lead to process improvement that benefits both quality and patient safety.

Table 1: Comparison Table – UKAS vs MHRA

Aspect	UKAS	MHRA

Full Name	United Kingdom Accreditation Service	Medicines and Healthcare products Regulatory Agency
Main-Focus	Quality and competence of laboratory services	Safety, quality, and regulatory compliance of blood, medicines, and medical devices
Applicable Standards	ISO15189 (Medical laboratories - Quality and competence)	Blood Safety and Quality Regulations (BSQR 2005)
Scope	All pathology disciplines - Haematology, Biochemistry, Microbiology, Histopathology, etc.	Mainly Blood Transfusion and any use of medicines or medical devices
Inspections Include	Document control, IQC/EQA performance, training records, SOP compliance, audits	Traceability of blood, cold chain, incident reporting (SABRE), equipment validation
Outcome of Visit	Accreditation decision and non-conformance reports with CAPA submission	Regulatory compliance report and follow-up actions to maintain BSQR standards
Examples	Checking analyser maintenance logs in Biochemistry, or competency files in Haematology	Reviewing blood fridge temperature logs and SABRE incident reports in Transfusion
Goal	Ensure reliable, accurate, and consistent laboratory testing	Ensure patient safety and legal compliance in handling blood and medicines

Summary:

UKAS focuses on quality and competence, accrediting laboratories to ISO15189 standards, while MHRA focuses on regulatory compliance and the safety and traceability of blood and medical products. Both are essential in ensuring that laboratories deliver accurate, reliable, and safe results. As a Biomedical Scientist, understanding and applying the requirements of both bodies such as maintaining traceability, documentation, equipment calibration, and corrective actions helps uphold the laboratory's integrity and ensure patient safety.

Question 98:

Can you tell us the two or three things you have done that you are proud of.

Background:

This question is designed to test your self-awareness, motivation, and professional achievements. In laboratory practice, being "proud" of something often reflects your contribution to quality improvement, patient safety, teamwork, or personal development. The interviewers want to know what you value most in your work, how you measure success, and how your achievements align with the organisation's goals and values.

Points to consider:

- Choose examples that demonstrate professional growth, initiative, and contribution to the team or laboratory.
- Include achievements that reflect technical competence, leadership, or improvement of service quality.
- Provide clear outcomes - how your actions benefitted the laboratory, staff, or patient care.
- Use practical examples to support your answer.

Answer:

There are a few things I am particularly proud of in my career as a Biomedical Scientist because they reflect my passion for quality, learning, and teamwork.

1. **Improving Turnaround Time in Biochemistry:**

While working **in the Biochemistry department**, I noticed delays in processing urgent (STAT) samples during peak hours. I collaborated with colleagues to review the workflow and suggested reallocating staff temporarily to the centrifugation area during busy periods. This reduced waiting time and improved turnaround time (TAT) for urgent tests by almost 20%. I was proud because this improvement directly supported faster diagnosis and patient management, which is at the heart of laboratory work.

2. **Supporting a Junior Colleague to Achieve Competence:**

In Haematology, I mentored a newly qualified Band 5 scientist who initially struggled with analyser troubleshooting and result validation. I took time to train them, using real examples from daily bench work and explaining the reasoning behind each decision. Within a few months, the colleague gained full competency and confidence. I was proud of this because it showed the value of teamwork, knowledge sharing, and supporting others to succeed, which is one of the key principles in maintaining a strong laboratory team.

3. **Ensuring Full Compliance During an MHRA Inspection:**

While working **in Blood Transfusion**, I helped prepare the department for an upcoming MHRA inspection by reviewing documentation, ensuring fridge logs and training records were up to date, and verifying traceability records. During the inspection, there were no critical findings, and the inspector commended our team for excellent traccability compliance. I was particularly proud of this because it reflected our collective commitment to patient safety and regulatory compliance.

Summary:

I am proud of the progress I have made as a Biomedical Scientist and how my work has contributed to patient care and service improvement. For example, I helped improve turnaround times by reviewing and suggesting small process changes on the bench, supported colleagues by sharing knowledge during training sessions, and followed quality procedures that ensured compliance with UKAS and MHRA standards. These experiences have helped me grow in confidence, strengthen my technical and communication skills, and understand the importance of teamwork and accuracy in maintaining laboratory quality and patient safety.

Question 99:

How do you train a junior staff?

Background:

Training junior staff is one of the core responsibilities in the pathology laboratory. The goal is to help new or less experienced colleagues gain competence and confidence in performing their duties safely and accurately. The training process must align with the department's Standard Operating Procedures (SOPs) and ISO15189 standards. Effective training ensures consistency, maintains laboratory quality, and supports staff development. This question tests your ability to mentor, assess competency, and communicate effectively while ensuring patient safety is never compromised.

Points to consider:

- Importance of structured and continuous training in the laboratory.
- Understanding that training supports competency, confidence, and staff integration.
- Link to ISO15189, SOP, and Quality Management System (QMS).

- Encourage a supportive learning environment with constructive feedback.
- Use examples to support your answer.

Answer:

Training junior staff requires a structured, patient, and hands-on approach that supports their gradual development in both technical and professional aspects. For me I usually start by welcoming the staff and helping them integrate into the team. For example, introducing them to colleagues, explaining lab safety rules, and showing them essential areas such as the staff room, specimen reception, and analyser benches. This builds confidence and a sense of belonging.

Next, I ensure the new staff member has access to Q-Pulse (or the laboratory document control system) to review key SOPs, policies, and competency documents relevant to their section. I encourage them to read and ask questions to build theoretical understanding before hands-on training.

Once someone is comfortable with the basics, I demonstrate bench procedures step by step, explaining the reasoning behind each action. I believe strongly in learning by example, so that understanding extends beyond *how* a task is performed to *why* it is done in a particular way. In Haematology, for instance, this might involve showing how to run and interpret daily quality control on an analyser before supervising as the process is repeated. In Blood Transfusion, it includes demonstrating correct sample labelling and handling to minimise the risk of patient identification errors.

As confidence develops, I observe junior colleagues carrying out the task under supervision, using any mistakes or uncertainties as opportunities for learning rather than criticism. Feedback is constructive and always linked back to the relevant procedure. Once competence is consistently demonstrated, supervision is gradually reduced until the individual is able to work independently, safely, and with confidence.

When they reach that stage, I assign competency assessments, review their evidence, and sign off only when confident in their ability. For example, **in Biochemistry**, a trainee may progress from loading samples on the analyser to performing calibration, reviewing QC, and validating results once trained and competent.

Additionally, I encourage continuous learning through CPD, case discussions, and reflective practice to reinforce knowledge and confidence.

Summary:

I train junior staff through a structured, step-by-step process: orientation, theory, demonstration, supervised practice, and competency assessment. My approach focuses on building confidence, competence, and adherence to SOPs while maintaining a supportive learning environment. For example, in Blood Transfusion, I ensure a junior colleague practices safe sample handling and crossmatch procedures under close supervision until they can perform independently. This method not only enhances their technical skills but also strengthens laboratory teamwork and ensures patient safety aligning with ISO15189 and QMS principles.

Question 100:

Take us through your education and experience.

Background:

This moment offers an opportunity to reflect on a professional journey and to show how education and experience come together in practice. It highlights the progression from academic foundations to hands-on laboratory training, and how each stage builds the knowledge, skills, and judgement required of a Biomedical Scientist.

It also speaks to alignment. Different laboratory disciplines demand different strengths, and understanding how one's background fits within areas such as Haematology, Blood Transfusion,

Biochemistry, Microbiology, or Histopathology helps illustrate both professional growth and readiness to contribute meaningfully to a specific department.

Points to consider:

- Summarise your academic background relevant to Biomedical Science.
- Include key qualifications (e.g., BSc Biomedical Science, HCPC registration, IBMS registration portfolio, MSc if applicable).
- Highlight your practical experience, training placements, and previous job roles.
- Link your education and experience to the department and job role.
- Mention any transferable skills gained from non-laboratory work (e.g., healthcare assistant, cleaner, phlebotomist, medical lab assistant).
- Use examples to demonstrate how your learning and experience have prepared you for the Biomedical Scientist position.

Answer:

I began my academic journey with a BSc (Hons) in Biomedical Science, which provided me with a strong theoretical understanding of human biology, pathophysiology, and laboratory diagnostics. During my degree, I studied key modules such as Clinical Biochemistry, Haematology, Blood Transfusion, Medical Microbiology, and Histopathology, all of which gave me a broad foundation in laboratory science and quality assurance.

As part of my degree, I completed an IBMS-accredited placement year in an NHS pathology laboratory. During that time, I gained hands-on experience in sample reception, analyser operation, internal quality control (IQC), and interpreting results under supervision. For example, **in Haematology**, I became familiar with full blood count analysis, troubleshooting flags such as atypical lymphocytes, and performing manual differentials when required. **In Blood Transfusion**, I was trained on safe sample labelling such as recommended five identifies, antibody screening, crossmatching, and issuing blood components using the LIMS.

After graduation, I completed my IBMS Registration Training Portfolio, which allowed me to demonstrate competence across all key laboratory disciplines in line with HCPC standards of proficiency. Once my portfolio was verified, I achieved HCPC registration as a Biomedical Scientist.

In my current role, I work in Biochemistry, where my days are shaped by a balance of routine and urgent work. I analyse samples, monitor internal and external quality control, validate patient results, and help troubleshoot analyser issues as they arise. During periods of particularly high workload, I have learned the importance of prioritisation and teamwork, ensuring that urgent requests are processed promptly while routine work continues to flow smoothly.

Beyond the laboratory bench, my earlier roles within healthcare gave me a broader understanding of how each part of the system connects. Working in positions such as healthcare assistant, medical laboratory assistant, and cleaner deepened my appreciation of infection control, patient care, and the often unseen value of multidisciplinary teamwork. These experiences continue to shape how I approach my work in the laboratory, with respect for every role involved in delivering safe and effective patient care.

I continue to develop professionally through CPD activities, including online IBMS webinars, internal training, and participation in audit and quality improvement initiatives by ensuring my knowledge stays up to date with modern laboratory practices.

Summary:

My educational background in Biomedical Science and my practical experience in various laboratory settings have prepared me to work confidently and competently as a Biomedical Scientist. My academic training gave me a strong scientific foundation, while my hands-on experience from my student placement to registered practice taught me accuracy,

teamwork, and accountability. I believe this combination of theory, practice, and continuous learning makes me well-equipped to contribute effectively to patient-centred laboratory service delivery.

Question 101:

What current training have you done?

Background:

Continuous professional development (CPD) and ongoing training are essential in pathology laboratories to maintain competence, ensure accuracy, and comply with professional and regulatory standards such as ISO 15189, UKAS, and HCPC. Biomedical Scientists are expected to engage in structured learning through mandatory, departmental, and external training to enhance their knowledge and uphold patient safety. This question evaluates your understanding of the importance of ongoing training, your commitment to continued learning, and how your recent training has contributed to laboratory quality and effective service delivery.

Points to Consider:

- Importance of continuous training and lifelong learning.
- Compliance with ISO 15189, UKAS, and HCPC CPD requirements.
- Examples of recent training (departmental and mandatory).
- Impact of the training on competence, service improvement, and patient safety.
- Application of knowledge gained from training.

Answer:

Continuous training is a key part of maintaining competence and ensuring the quality of results produced in the laboratory. I take part in various forms of training such as mandatory, technical, specialist, and reflective training, which helped me to ensure I stay updated both professionally and technically.

In Biochemistry, I recently completed training on the installation and validation of a new clinical chemistry analyser, which involved verification studies, calibration, precision testing, and comparison with the previous analyser to ensure consistent performance. This experience improved my understanding of equipment validation in line with ISO 15189 standards.

In Haematology, I attended in-house blood film morphology refresher sessions, focusing on identifying key abnormal cells such as blasts, schistocytes, and spherocytes. This helped me strengthen my interpretative and reporting confidence, particularly in complex cases.

In Blood Transfusion, I completed traceability and major haemorrhage protocol (MHP) refresher training, where I learned updated procedures on managing emergency blood requests and the correct documentation for traceability compliance with MHRA regulations.

In Microbiology, I participated in training related to antimicrobial susceptibility testing (AST) and the interpretation of zone diameters using EUCAST guidelines. This reinforced my ability to identify resistance patterns and communicate critical results promptly.

In Histopathology, I completed specimen reception and embedding training, ensuring correct tissue orientation and documentation for diagnostic accuracy. The training emphasised the importance of sample traceability and pre-analytical quality control.

Alongside departmental training, I also complete Trust-wide mandatory training such as Health and Safety, Fire Safety, Equality, Diversity and Inclusion (EDI), Data Protection, and Safeguarding. These courses ensure I consistently maintain safe practice and professional conduct across all aspects of my work.

I also maintain a CPD log through my HCPC portfolio, recording all training, workshops, and reflective practices. This ensures I meet the professional requirements for revalidation and demonstrate continual improvement in my practice.

Summary:

I am committed to continuous professional development and regularly engage in both technical and mandatory training to maintain competence and compliance with regulatory standards. Through recent training in analyser validation, blood film morphology, traceability, AST interpretation, and tissue embedding, I have improved my technical and analytical skills across multiple disciplines. These experiences have not only enhanced my personal competence but also contributed to maintaining high laboratory standards, patient safety, and service efficiency.

Question 102:

What makes you the best candidate for the job?

Background:

This question assesses how well your skills, knowledge, and values align with the job description and person specification for the advertised Biomedical Scientist role. Interviewers use it to determine whether you understand the expectations of the position, can demonstrate competence through relevant experience, and will integrate effectively within the department and Trust culture. Biomedical Scientists are expected to demonstrate technical accuracy, strong quality awareness, effective teamwork, ongoing professional development, and a patient-focused approach, in line with ISO 15189, MHRA, and HCPC standards.

Points to Consider:

- Refer to the person specification (education, skills, experience, and values). See example in Table 2.
- Link your technical and soft skills to job expectations.
- Demonstrate teamwork, initiative, and problem-solving abilities.

- Use practical, evidence-based examples from multiple departments.
- Align your response with Trust values (e.g., compassion, accountability, integrity, improvement).

Table 2: Person of Specification Breakdown Example (For BMS role – may differ from role to role):

Specification Area	Example of Alignment
Qualification	Registered Biomedical Scientist with HCPC; BSc in Biomedical Science; IBMS Specialist Portfolio in progress or completed.
Experience	Demonstrated competence across multiple disciplines such as Haematology, Biochemistry, Blood Transfusion, or Microbiology. Experience in quality systems and analyser operation.
Knowledge and Skills	Knowledge of ISO 15189, UKAS audits, EQA/IQA, SOP compliance, analyser troubleshooting, and validation. Skilled in using LIMS and handling urgent samples.
Personal Qualities	Team player, proactive, good communicator, adaptable, and committed to patient safety and service improvement.
Trust Values Alignment	Compassionate care, integrity, teamwork, and continuous improvement reflected in daily practice and interactions.

Answer:

I believe I am the best candidate for this role because my qualifications, experience, and professional values directly align with the person specification and the Trust's commitment to providing high-quality, patient-focused laboratory services.

From the person specification, I understand that the role requires technical competence, adherence to quality systems, and the ability to work effectively both independently and as part of a team. Throughout my career, I have demonstrated these consistently.

For example, **in Haematology,** I identified an opportunity to improve turnaround times during peak hours by helping to reorganise the workflow and prioritisation of urgent samples. This improved TAT and maintained quality, which fulfilled the specification requirement for analytical efficiency and problem-solving.

In Biochemistry, I was part of a verification team for a new analyser. I participated in the precision and correlation testing phase and helped document the validation report in line with ISO 15189 standards. This demonstrated both technical ability and attention to quality documentation.

In Blood Transfusion, I have handled high-pressure situations such as major haemorrhage protocols. I ensured all crossmatches, compatibility checks, and documentation were accurate and that traceability requirements set by MHRA were strictly followed. This demonstrated accountability, confidence, and calmness under pressure, which is key traits for a BMS.

Beyond technical skills, I value collaboration and mentorship. I have supported the training of Band 5 scientists, guiding them through SOPs and competency assessments. This reflects my communication and leadership ability, which are essential soft skills in the person specification.

Additionally, I regularly engage in CPD activities, including internal training, webinars on analytical performance, and national scientific meetings. This ensures I stay updated with emerging technologies and regulatory changes, reinforcing professional growth and compliance with HCPC standards.

Summary:

I believe I am the best candidate for this position because I meet and exceed the key person specification areas such as technical competence, quality focus, teamwork, and professional development. My hands-on experience across Haematology, Biochemistry, and Blood Transfusion, combined with a proactive approach to training, quality improvement, and patient care, has prepared me to contribute effectively from day one. I am motivated by excellence, work consistently in line with SOPs, and remain focused on delivering accurate, timely, and safe results to support patient wellbeing.

Question 103:

Why choose to work here or the Trust?

Background:

Every NHS Trust has its own culture, structure, and service priorities. Although laboratory standards across the UK are governed by ISO 15189, UKAS, and HCPC requirements, the way a Trust delivers its pathology services can differ. For example, through specialisation (e.g., transfusion, molecular, or microbiology focus), the size of its catchment area, or its partnership with other hospitals. This question tests whether you've researched the Trust, understand its values and service model, and can explain how your skills, passion, and career goals align with what the Trust offers.

Points to Consider:

- Mention that each Trust has its own structure, values, and service priorities.
- Highlight why this Trust in particular appeals to you - reputation, facilities, opportunities, or specialties.
- Align your answer with the Trust values (e.g., compassion, teamwork, excellence, respect).

- Show understanding of how your experience fits into their service model.
- Give practical examples of how you would contribute to the Trust's goals.

Answer:

Every Trust has its own unique structure and priorities, even though all operate under the same regulatory standards as ISO 15189, UKAS, HTA, and MHRA etc. What attracted me to this Trust is its strong reputation for quality improvement, staff development, and patient-centred laboratory services.

For example, the Trust's focus on integrated pathology networks and cross-site collaboration reflects a commitment to innovation and efficiency that I value highly. Having previously worked in a multi-site setting, I understand how essential clear communication and harmonised SOPs are in maintaining consistent standards and ensuring seamless service delivery across departments.

I am also drawn to the Trust's commitment to continuous professional development (CPD) and staff training. I believe in lifelong learning and have regularly undertaken CPD activities such as internal competency assessments, participation in EQA reviews, and attending IBMS-accredited workshops. Joining a Trust that prioritises staff development means I can continue to grow professionally while contributing my experience to mentor others.

From a service perspective, the Trust's use of modern automated systems and digital LIMS integration aligns with my technical background. For example, in my previous role, I helped validate a new analyser interface to improve result accuracy and turnaround time, which is a skill that would directly support this Trust's focus on service efficiency and patient safety.

I also appreciate the Trust's values of compassion, accountability, and teamwork, which align closely with my personal approach to laboratory work by ensuring every sample is treated with the same care and urgency as if it belonged to a family member.

Summary:

I chose this Trust because of its commitment to quality, innovation, and staff development, and because its values align with my own professional principles. While every Trust operates differently, this one's emphasis on teamwork, patient-centred service, and continuous improvement perfectly matches my experience and goals. I am confident that I can contribute to its mission of delivering safe, accurate, and timely laboratory results that support the best possible patient care.

Please see below practical Examples from three different Trust – Use it as a Template (Research specific – about the Trust you are attending the interview):

Example 1: Manchester University NHS Foundation Trust (MFT)

Answer:

Each Trust has its own strengths and focused areas, and what drew me to Manchester University NHS Foundation Trust is its reputation for innovation, teaching, and research excellence. As one of the largest NHS Trusts in the UK, MFT offers exposure to a wide range of pathology disciplines, which provides opportunities to develop expertise across specialties.

MFT's investment in modern automation systems and its leading role within the Greater Manchester Pathology Network align strongly with my interest in quality improvement and operational efficiency. In my current role, I supported the verification of a new analyser interface, which helped improve turnaround times for urgent biochemistry tests. This experience has strengthened my understanding of service optimisation, and it is something I would be keen to bring to this Trust.

Furthermore, I value the Trust's commitment to staff development and CPD. MFT's structured approach to continuous learning fits perfectly with my goal of completing my Specialist Portfolio and eventually progressing to senior roles.

Summary:

I chose MFT because of its scale, innovation, and culture of learning. These values mirror my passion for quality, development, and delivering excellent patient care in a modern, research-driven environment.

Example 2: Nottingham University Hospitals NHS Trust (NUH)

Answer:

Nottingham University Hospitals NHS Trust stands out for its strong commitment to education, research, and patient-centred care. As part of a major teaching hospital network, the Trust's laboratories manage a diverse range of cases and complex diagnostic challenges. This is exactly the kind of environment in which I believe I would thrive, allowing me to develop professionally while contributing meaningfully to high-quality patient care.

I am particularly impressed by NUH's role in the East Midlands Pathology Network and its commitment to continuous improvement through quality management systems. In my previous role, I contributed to a quality audit that improved sample handling efficiency, ensuring better compliance with ISO 15189.

NUH also promotes staff engagement and professional development, encouraging staff to pursue further education and CPD. As someone who regularly updates my competencies through EQA reviews, internal audits, and attending pathology conferences, I believe my drive for improvement aligns well with NUH's culture.

Summary:

I am drawn to NUH because it combines high professional standards with a supportive learning environment. I believe my technical background, quality focus, and teamwork skills will enable me to contribute effectively to the Trust's mission of delivering safe and high-quality laboratory services.

Example 3: Royal Free London NHS Foundation Trust (RFL)

Answer:

Royal Free London NHS Foundation Trust has an outstanding reputation for clinical excellence, research, and innovation. The Trust's laboratories serve a wide population and support several specialist services, including liver transplantation and infectious disease diagnostics. These are areas I find both challenging and rewarding.

I admire RFL's commitment to developing staff through structured training and mentorship, which reflects my belief in lifelong learning and professional growth. I have experience mentoring junior colleagues and training staff through competency assessments, which I can bring to this role.

RFL's value of "working together for patients" strongly aligns with my own practice. For example, I have worked closely with clinicians and nurses to clarify urgent test results, ensuring patient safety and timely treatment decisions, which is an approach that fits the Trust's collaborative ethos.

Summary:

I chose RFL because of its strong patient focus, research excellence, and investment in staff development. I believe I can contribute to the Trust's mission through my technical expertise, teamwork, and dedication to maintaining high laboratory standards.

Question 104:

What are the functions of a Blood Sciences Laboratory?

Background:

The Blood Sciences Laboratory is a core component of Pathology, integrating several key diagnostic disciplines, including Haematology, Clinical Biochemistry, Immunology, and Blood Transfusion. It plays a vital role in supporting patient diagnosis, monitoring treatment, and aiding disease prevention. This question assesses your understanding of the scope and function of the Blood Sciences Laboratory, as well as your ability to relate these functions to patient care, effective service delivery, and multidisciplinary teamwork, in line with ISO 15189 and other relevant professional standards.

Points to Consider:

- Define what "Blood Sciences" encompasses.
- Discuss the core functions of the Blood Sciences Laboratory.
- Mention examples of tests performed and clinical relevance.
- Refer to quality assurance, automation, and accreditation standards.
- Highlight teamwork, data integrity, and communication with clinicians.
- Use examples across departments to show comprehensive understanding.

Answer:

The Blood Sciences Laboratory is a central component of pathology that combines several disciplines, which are: Haematology, Clinical Biochemistry, Immunology, and Blood Transfusion. Each of these departments collaboratively work together to provide accurate, timely, and reliable diagnostic information that directly supports patient care.

Let us see few examples as shown below:

Haematology:

Haematology focuses on the study of blood and its components such as red cells, white cells, and platelets. The laboratory performs tests such as full blood counts (FBC), blood film morphology, coagulation profiles, and haemoglobin electrophoresis to diagnose and monitor conditions like anaemia, leukaemia, clotting disorders, and infections.

For example, during an emergency case such as suspected deep vein thrombosis, rapid coagulation testing (PT, APTT, D-dimer) helps clinicians make timely decisions regarding anticoagulant therapy.

Clinical Biochemistry:

Clinical Biochemistry analyses body fluids (e.g. serum, plasma, urine) to evaluate organ function and monitor metabolic processes. Common tests include renal, liver, cardiac, lipid, and electrolyte profiles.

For example, during a myocardial infarction (heart attack), urgent troponin levels are measured to guide clinical management. Automation and advanced analysers is central to enable the lab process high sample volumes efficiently while maintaining result accuracy in blood sciences.

Immunology:

The Immunology section detects and measures antibodies, antigens, and immune complexes, helping diagnose autoimmune diseases, allergies, and immune deficiencies. Tests such as antinuclear antibody (ANA), rheumatoid factor (RF), and thyroid antibodies support clinicians in managing autoimmune thyroid disease or rheumatoid arthritis.

Blood Transfusion:

This section is responsible for ensuring the safe and compatible provision of blood and blood components to patients. It includes activities such as blood grouping, antibody screening, crossmatching, and the issuing of units for both elective surgeries and emergency situations, including major haemorrhage protocols (MHP).

For example, when a trauma patient requires urgent transfusion, the Blood Transfusion team must act rapidly to verify patient identification, perform appropriate compatibility testing or electronic issue, and ensure the correct units are supplied to prevent transfusion reactions and support safe patient outcomes.

Other Core Functions:

Quality Assurance and Accreditation:

The laboratory operates under strict quality systems guided by ISO 15189 to ensure accuracy, reproducibility, and traceability of results. Internal Quality Control (IQC) and External Quality Assessment (EQA) schemes verify analytical performance.

Equipment Maintenance and Verification:

Regular analyser calibration, maintenance, and validation of new equipment or methods ensure consistency and reliability of test results.

Clinical Communication and Interpretation:

Biomedical Scientists work closely with clinicians to provide interpretive comments on results and ensure that urgent or abnormal results are promptly communicated to the clinicians, which contribute to supporting timely patient management.

Training and Development:

The laboratory supports CPD, portfolio completion, and competency assessment of staff to maintain a skilled workforce that delivers safe and effective service.

Summary:

The Blood Sciences Laboratory performs a wide range of diagnostic tests across Haematology, Biochemistry, Immunology, and Transfusion Science, which are all essential to patient diagnosis, treatment, and monitoring. Its core functions include accurate testing, quality assurance, equipment management, and multidisciplinary collaboration. Through automation, adherence to ISO 15189, and effective teamwork, Blood Sciences ensures the delivery of timely, accurate, and reliable results that directly support patient safety and clinical decision-making.

Question 105:

What are the skills you have to function in this role?

Background:

The role of a Biomedical Scientist (BMS) requires a broad mix of technical, analytical, interpersonal, and organisational skills. These skills ensure that laboratory work is accurate, efficient, and compliant with regulatory standards like ISO 15189, UKAS, and MHRA. This question tests your self-awareness and understanding of the key competencies needed to perform effectively within a Blood Sciences laboratory or similar diagnostic setting. It also gives you a chance to demonstrate how your personal strengths align with the job description and person specification of the role you're applying for.

Points to Consider:

- Highlight technical, analytical, communication, and IT skills relevant to laboratory practice.
- Demonstrate understanding of quality management and compliance.
- Include teamwork, problem solving, and time management skills.

- Relate your skills to the person specification of the advertised role.
- Provide practical examples where appropriate - across disciplines (Haematology, Biochemistry, Transfusion, Histopathology, Microbiology).

Answer:

To function effectively as a Biomedical Scientist, I have developed a wide range of technical, analytical, and interpersonal skills that enable me to deliver high-quality results and maintain patient safety.

Technical and Analytical Skills:

I have strong analytical and problem-solving skills that enable me to interpret complex results accurately. For example, **in Haematology**, I can review abnormal blood film findings and correlate them with FBC results, while **in Biochemistry**, I am confident in validating abnormal electrolyte results by assessing sample integrity and patient history. I also have extensive hands-on experience in operating, maintaining, and troubleshooting automated analysers such as Sysmex, Roche Cobas, and Abbott Alinity systems and ensuring smooth laboratory operations.

Quality and Compliance Awareness:

I have a sound understanding of ISO 15189 standards, UKAS accreditation requirements, HTA, and MHRA guidelines, which are used to guide daily practice in maintaining laboratory quality. For example, when performing internal quality control (IQC) or reviewing EQA results, I ensure that any deviation from the expected range is properly documented, investigated, and corrective action taken to prevent reoccurrence.

IT and Data Management Skills:

I am proficient in using Laboratory Information Management Systems (LIMS) such as WinPath, MediTech, LabCentre, Telepath, Cerna, Bank Manager and Clinisys, which ensures accurate data entry, result validation, and traceability. I also use IT tools such as

Excel and laboratory middleware to monitor trends in QC performance and generate audit reports, which are essential for continuous improvement.

Communication and Teamwork Skills:

Effective communication is vital in the laboratory environment. I regularly liaise with colleagues, clinicians, and nurses to clarify sample or result discrepancies. For example, **in Blood Transfusion**, if a sample fails compatibility checks, I promptly contact the ward, verify patient identifiers, and explain the need for a repeat sample to ensure transfusion safety. I also contribute positively to teamwork by supporting colleagues during analyser downtime or helping new staff understand workflow processes.

Time Management and Prioritisation Skills:

Working in a fast-paced environment such as Blood Sciences requires the ability to prioritise. For example, during out-of-hours shifts, I manage urgent A&E, ITU, and major haemorrhage requests efficiently while maintaining turnaround times for routine samples.

Training and Mentoring Skills:

I enjoy supporting junior staff and students through training and competency assessment. I provide practical demonstrations and feedback to help them meet laboratory standards and understand the clinical relevance of their work.

Adaptability and Continuous Learning:

Pathology is a continually evolving field, and I ensure my knowledge remains up to date through CPD activities, internal training sessions, and relevant professional courses. For example, I recently completed a course on laboratory automation and data integrity, which has strengthened my understanding of efficiency, compliance, and the effective use of digital systems within the laboratory

Summary:

I possess a balanced combination of technical, analytical, communication, and leadership skills that enable me to function effectively as a Biomedical Scientist. My experience in quality assurance, equipment maintenance, data management, and team collaboration aligns well with the person specification for this role. I believe my skills not only support accurate and timely patient results but also contribute to continuous improvement and the overall success of the laboratory service.

Question 106:

How do you approach work, bearing in mind flexibility?

Background:

Biomedical Scientists and other laboratory staff work in dynamic environments where workload, sample type, and staffing levels can vary significantly. Flexibility is essential to maintain service quality, patient safety, and timely reporting of results. This question tests your understanding of adaptability, prioritisation, and teamwork in laboratory practice.

Points to Consider:

- Demonstrate understanding of dynamic workload in labs.
- Show ability to prioritise urgent tasks while maintaining routine work.
- Highlight teamwork, adaptability, and problem-solving skills.
- Include practical examples across departments.
- Mention readiness to adapt to shift patterns, new equipment, or processes.

Answer:

I approach work with a combination of organisation, adaptability, and clear prioritisation. Flexibility is a key aspect of laboratory work because unexpected situations arise regularly, such as urgent clinical samples, equipment downtime, or staff shortages.

For example, **in Biochemistry**, if a critical electrolyte panel for an ICU patient arrives while routine samples are being processed, I will pause routine work and prioritise the urgent sample to ensure patient care is not compromised, then return to routine tasks to maintain turnaround times.

In Blood Transfusion, flexibility is essential. During a major haemorrhage, I may need to temporarily step away from routine crossmatches to handle urgent blood product requests, ensuring I follow SOPs while coordinating with colleagues for support in non-urgent tasks.

In Haematology, I have adapted to situations where the analyser is down by manually preparing and running critical samples while maintaining accurate records, and liaising with the senior team to ensure continuity of service.

Flexibility also involves adapting to new equipment, updated SOPs, or policy changes. For example, when a new analyser or reagent batch is introduced, I adjust my workflow to accommodate verification and validation tasks without disrupting other lab operations.

Summary:

I approach work with organisation, prioritisation, and adaptability, ensuring urgent tasks are addressed without neglecting routine responsibilities. Flexibility allows me to respond effectively to unexpected situations such as urgent patient samples, staff shortages, or equipment issues, while maintaining SOP compliance and patient safety. By balancing routine work with unexpected demands, I ensure consistent quality across all laboratory services, demonstrating both reliability and resilience as a Biomedical Scientist.

Question 107:

What is patient confidentiality, data protection and the legislation governing it?

Background:

Patient confidentiality is fundamental to healthcare and laboratory practice, ensuring that personal and medical information is kept private and only shared with authorised personnel. Data protection refers to the legal and organisational measures in place to safeguard personal data from misuse, loss, or unauthorised access. This question assesses your understanding of the ethical and legal responsibilities involved in handling patient information, in line with relevant legislation such as the Data Protection Act 2018 and UK GDPR, as well as professional guidance from the HCPC, UKAS, and NHS policies.

Points to Consider:

- Define patient confidentiality and why it is important.
- Define data protection and its relevance in the lab.
- Mention legislation that governs handling of patient information (e.g., Data Protection Act 2018, UK GDPR).
- Give practical examples of how confidentiality and data protection are maintained in laboratory practice.
- Highlight consequences of breaches to patient safety, ethics, or legal compliance.

Answer:

Patient confidentiality means ensuring that any personal or medical information about a patient is kept private and only shared with authorised personnel who require it for the purpose of care or treatment. In the laboratory setting, this includes safeguarding test results, diagnostic information, and any identifiable patient details to ensure privacy and maintain trust in the healthcare system.

Data protection refers to the steps taken to secure patient information from unauthorised access, accidental loss, or misuse. In practice, this includes ensuring LIMS access is password-protected, reports are sent securely, and paper records are stored safely.

The key legislation governing confidentiality and data protection includes the UK General Data Protection Regulation (UK GDPR) and the Data Protection Act 2018. These outline patients' rights over their personal data, the responsibilities of healthcare providers, and the potential consequences of breaches. In addition, professional guidance from the HCPC, UKAS, MHRA, and NHS policies further reinforces how confidential information should be managed within laboratory settings to ensure compliance and protect patient privacy.

Practical examples:

- **In Biochemistry,** I ensure that when emailing critical results to a ward, the correct patient identifiers are used, and the email is secure.

- **In Haematology,** patient labels are checked carefully before reporting results to prevent releasing information for the wrong patient.

- **In Histopathology,** slides and reports are stored securely in restricted areas, ensuring only authorised personnel have access.

- I also avoid discussing patient results in public areas and train junior staff on confidentiality in line with SOPs.

Summary:

Patient confidentiality and data protection are about safeguarding patient information and sharing it only with those who are authorised. Compliance with the Data Protection Act 2018, UK GDPR, and professional guidance ensures legal and ethical practice. In the laboratory, I apply these principles by securely handling samples and results, restricting access to patient data, and mentoring junior staff. Protecting patient information maintains trust, ethical standards, and safety across all pathology services.

Question 108:

What is QMS and Tools used in QMS?

Background:

A Quality Management System (QMS) is a structured framework that ensures a laboratory consistently delivers high-quality, accurate, and reliable results in line with international standards such as ISO15189. It provides policies, procedures, and practices to monitor, evaluate, and improve laboratory performance. This question tests your understanding of how QMS supports laboratory quality, patient safety, and compliance, as well as your knowledge of practical tools used within QMS to maintain standards.

Points to Consider:

- Define QMS in simple terms.
- Explain importance of QMS in pathology laboratories.
- Identify tools and mechanisms used in QMS.
- Link QMS to ISO15189 and patient safety.
- Provide practical examples across different lab departments.

Answer:

A Quality Management System (QMS) is a framework of policies, procedures, and processes designed to ensure the laboratory delivers accurate, reliable, and timely results. It focuses on maintaining standards, preventing errors, and improving performance to ensure patient safety and regulatory compliance.

Tools used in QMS include:

- **Standard Operating Procedures (SOPs):** Detailed instructions for every task to ensure consistency. For example, **in Biochemistry**, SOPs outline how to run and validate analysers.

- **Internal Audits:** Regular checks to assess compliance with SOPs and ISO15189 standards. **In Haematology**, audits may focus on sample handling and labelling.

- **External Quality Assessment (EQA):** Participation in schemes to benchmark lab performance against peers. For example, **a Microbiology lab** may use EQA to validate pathogen identification accuracy.

- **Corrective and Preventive Actions (CAPA):** Used to investigate and resolve non-conformances. **In Blood Transfusion,** a near-miss in blood crossmatch would trigger CAPA.

- **Training and Competency Records:** Ensuring staff are competent to perform procedures. For example, **Histopathology** staff undergo training on tissue processing and slide preparation.

- **Calibration and Maintenance Logs:** For equipment performance monitoring. For example, analysers **in Biochemistry** are routinely calibrated and maintained with records kept in the QMS.

- **Document Control and Change Management:** Ensuring all policies, SOPs, and forms are up-to-date and authorised.

These tools collectively ensure the laboratory meets ISO15189 standards, prevents errors, and maintains consistent quality across all analytical, pre-analytical, and post-analytical processes.

Summary:

A QMS is a structured system that ensures laboratory results are accurate, reliable, and compliant with standards. Tools such as SOPs, audits, EQA, CAPA, competency records, and calibration logs help maintain high-quality services. In practice, I apply QMS by following SOPs precisely, participating in audits and EQA schemes, logging equipment maintenance, and training colleagues, which collectively support patient safety and continuous improvement.

Question 109:

Laboratories in the UK are assessed by which external bodies? Name others.

Background:

Laboratories in the UK are subject to external assessment to ensure compliance with national and international standards. These assessments safeguard quality, patient safety, and regulatory compliance. This question evaluates your understanding of the key regulatory and accrediting bodies, as well as their roles in overseeing and maintaining the standards of laboratory services.

Points to Consider:

- Name the main external assessment bodies for UK laboratories.
- Mention other relevant regulatory or professional organisations.
- Explain the purpose of these bodies in maintaining laboratory quality.
- Give practical examples of how these assessments affect laboratory practice.

Answer:

In the UK, laboratories are assessed by several external bodies to ensure compliance with regulations and standards:

UKAS (United Kingdom Accreditation Service):

- Accredits laboratories against ISO15189, ensuring quality and competence.

- **Example:** A Biochemistry lab undergoing UKAS inspection will be assessed on equipment calibration, SOP adherence, and staff competency records.

MHRA (Medicines and Healthcare products Regulatory Agency):

- Regulates laboratories handling blood, tissues, and in-vitro diagnostic devices.

- **Example:** A Blood Transfusion lab will be inspected by MHRA for compliance with blood component handling and storage standards.

HTA (Human Tissue Authority):

- Regulates labs using human tissue for diagnostic or research purposes.

- **Example:** A Histopathology lab is inspected by HTA to ensure proper tissue consent, storage, and disposal practices.

RCPath (Royal College of Pathologists):

- Provides professional standards, guidelines, and audits for laboratory practice.

- **Example:** A Microbiology lab may follow RCPath guidelines on antimicrobial susceptibility testing and participate in peer review.

Other Bodies:

- **Care Quality Commission (CQC):** Inspects hospitals and laboratories for overall patient safety and care quality.

- **NHS Improvement or Trust Internal Audit Teams:** Conduct internal checks to determine alignment with national standards.

These external assessments help ensure patient safety, maintain high-quality laboratory services, and promote continuous improvement. Laboratories prepare for inspections by maintaining accurate documentation, conducting regular internal audits, and ensuring that staff remain competent and compliant with current standards.

Summary:

UK laboratories are primarily assessed by UKAS, MHRA, HTA, and RCPath, with additional oversight by bodies like CQC and internal audit teams. These external assessments ensure regulatory compliance, high-quality results, and patient safety. In practice, this means keeping accurate SOPs, competency records, and equipment logs, and participating in EQA schemes to meet standards across departments such as Biochemistry, Microbiology, Histopathology, and Blood Transfusion.

Question 110:

What is IQC and EQA, and their differences?

Background:

Maintaining laboratory accuracy and reliability is essential for patient safety and diagnostic confidence. Quality Control (QC) is an integral part of the Quality Management System (QMS) and is divided into Internal Quality Control (IQC) and External Quality Assessment (EQA). These systems ensure that laboratory results are accurate, reproducible, and consistent over time and between laboratories. This question assesses your understanding of both systems, their differences, and how they work together to support continuous quality improvement.

Points to Consider:

- Define IQC and EQA clearly.
- Explain the purpose of both and their importance in maintaining laboratory standards.
- Highlight key differences.
- Give practical examples where appropriate (e.g., Biochemistry, Haematology, Transfusion, Microbiology).
- Link to ISO15189 requirements.

Answer:

Internal Quality Control (IQC) and External Quality Assessment (EQA) are both essential tools used to ensure the reliability and accuracy of laboratory results (Table 3).

Internal Quality Control (IQC):

- IQC is a daily internal monitoring process that checks the accuracy and precision of results produced by the laboratory's analysers.

- It involves testing known control samples with established target ranges alongside patient samples to confirm that the analyser and reagents are performing correctly.

- IQC helps identify systematic or random errors before patient results are released.

Example:

In Biochemistry, IQC samples for analytes like sodium or glucose are run at least twice daily (morning and evening) to ensure analyser performance remains within acceptable limits. If a QC result falls outside the expected range, patient testing is stopped until the issue (e.g., reagent, calibration, or analyser fault) is resolved.

In Haematology, control samples for parameters like haemoglobin and platelet count are tested daily to monitor analyser stability and calibration accuracy.

External Quality Assessment (EQA):

- EQA is an independent external check where the laboratory receives unknown samples from an external provider (e.g., UK NEQAS).

- The samples are tested like patient samples, and the results are submitted to the EQA provider, who compares them against results from other participating laboratories.

- EQA assesses inter-laboratory accuracy and helps identify long-term trends or systematic errors.

Example:

In Blood Transfusion, EQA samples may be used to check antibody identification accuracy or compatibility testing procedures.

In Microbiology, EQA may involve identifying an unknown bacterial organism and reporting the correct antibiotic susceptibility profile.

Table 3: Key Differences Between IQC and EQA:

Feature	**IQC**	**EQA**
Frequency	Performed daily or per batch	Periodically (monthly or quarterly)
Purpose	Monitors analyser and process stability	Assesses lab performance compared to others
Sample Type	Known samples with expected ranges	Unknown samples from external provider
Scope	Internal, within the laboratory	External, across multiple laboratories
Responsibility	Managed by laboratory staff	Managed by an external quality provider (e.g., UK NEQAS)
Error Detection	Detects immediate analytical errors	Detects long-term systematic or procedural errors

Summary:

IQC and EQA are both critical components of laboratory quality assurance under ISO15189. IQC ensures the day-to-day accuracy and precision of results before release, while EQA ensures inter-laboratory comparability and long-term consistency. Together, they help maintain high-quality standards, build confidence in patient results, and promote continuous improvement across all laboratory disciplines such as Biochemistry and Haematology to Microbiology and Blood Transfusion.

Question 111:

What are the benefits of being open and honest when you make a mistake or error? What will you do when you make mistakes?

Background:

Mistakes can happen in any laboratory, regardless of experience or skill level. What differentiates a safe and professional laboratory from a risky one is how errors are handled. Being open and honest about mistakes supports the principles of duty of candour, patient safety, and continuous improvement. It ensures that errors are corrected quickly, lessons are learned, and systems are improved to prevent recurrence. This question tests your understanding of professional accountability, transparency, and your attitude towards learning from mistakes.

Points to Consider:

- Importance of honesty and transparency when errors occur.
- The concept of duty of candour and how it applies in the laboratory.
- Steps to take after identifying a mistake.
- How learning from errors improves personal and laboratory practice.
- Use of practical examples to demonstrate understanding.

Answer:

Being open and honest when a mistake occurs is fundamental to patient safety and professional integrity. It shows accountability, helps maintain trust, and allows corrective actions to be taken quickly to prevent harm or recurrence.

In the laboratory, transparency ensures that potential risks are addressed before they escalate. For example, if I realise that I validated the wrong patient's result due to similar names or sample mislabelling, I will immediately stop the process and escalate the issue to the senior biomedical scientist (BMS) or quality manager. I would also log the error on the incident management system (such as Datix or Q-Pulse) for proper investigation. The affected result would be corrected and rechecked before being released to the ward or clinician.

Being open about such errors helps determine whether the root cause is human error, a system failure, or a gap in existing processes. For example, if an error occurred because of unclear labelling, this may point to a pre-analytical issue that requires communication with nursing staff for clarification or retraining.

In Microbiology, if an incorrect sensitivity result was reported due to a misidentified organism, being transparent allows the lab to retract the result promptly, notify clinicians, and perform a root cause analysis to prevent similar occurrences.

Similarly, **in Blood Transfusion,** honesty is non-negotiable. For example, any potential discrepancy, such as incorrect blood group selection or crossmatch error, must be reported immediately to protect patient safety.

When I make a mistake, I follow a clear structure:

- **Acknowledge and stop** - Pause the process immediately.
- **Report** - Inform my senior or line manager as per SOP.

- **Investigate** - Participate in identifying the cause through the incident reporting process.

- **Reflect and learn** - Use reflective practice (CPD log) to understand what went wrong and how to avoid a repeat.

- **Share learning** - Contribute to departmental discussions or training sessions to help others learn from the event.

Summary:

Being open and honest about mistakes promotes a learning culture and upholds the principles of duty of candour. It ensures that corrective and preventive actions are taken quickly, protecting patient safety and enhancing professional development. By acknowledging mistakes, investigating causes, and sharing lessons learned, laboratory teams can continuously improve their systems and maintain public trust. For example, promptly reporting an incorrect validation, a mislabelled sample, or an analyser error not only resolves the issue but also strengthens the laboratory's commitment to quality and patient-centred care.

Question 112:

How do you cope as a lone worker in a high-pressured environment?

Background:

Working alone, especially in a high-pressure laboratory environment, requires a high level of competence, confidence, and effective time management. Lone working often occurs during out-of-hours (OOH) shifts, weekends, or in smaller departments. It tests your ability to prioritise tasks, remain calm under pressure, and know when to escalate for help. This question assesses your understanding of safe lone working practices, your ability to maintain quality and safety under stress, and how you manage workload while following established protocols.

Points to Consider:

- Understanding of lone working and its associated challenges.
- Awareness of standard operating procedures (SOPs) and risk assessments for lone working.
- Importance of communication, prioritisation, and knowing when to escalate.
- Use of realistic examples where applicable (e.g. Blood Transfusion, Biochemistry, Microbiology).
- Personal strategies to stay organised and calm.

Answer:

Coping as a lone worker in a high-pressure environment requires planning, composure, and a clear understanding of one's responsibilities and limitations. I ensure that I am familiar with the lone working policy and relevant SOPs, and that I know how to contact senior staff or on-call managers if required. For example, during out-of-hours (OOH) shifts **in Blood Transfusion**, I often work alone and must respond to urgent requests such as massive haemorrhage protocols (MHP) or emergency crossmatches. In such cases, I prioritise work based on clinical urgency. For example, ensuring that blood units for a bleeding patient are issued promptly while still maintaining accurate documentation and traceability. If multiple requests come at once, I contact the on-call biomedical scientist or duty manager for support or advice, ensuring that patient safety remains the top priority.

In Biochemistry, lone working might mean monitoring several analysers simultaneously. If one analyser goes down during a critical period, I stay calm, follow the downtime SOP, transfer urgent samples to a backup analyser if available, and inform the duty manager or service engineer.

Similarly, **in Microbiology,** working alone may involve prioritising urgent cultures or critical results (e.g. positive blood cultures). I would follow laboratory protocols to ensure timely communication to the clinical team, even while managing routine work.

Personally, I cope by staying organised in maintaining a clear workflow, avoiding distractions, and double-checking results before validation. I also take short mental breaks like stretching, deep breathing, and taking a short walk within the laboratory environment, when possible, to stay focused and reduce fatigue, particularly during long night shifts.

Summary:

Working as a lone worker in a high-pressured environment requires confidence, organisation, and sound judgement. I rely on my competence, adherence to SOPs, and effective communication with on-call support to ensure patient safety and service continuity. Staying calm, prioritising tasks, and seeking help when needed helps me maintain control and deliver accurate, timely results. For example, whether managing an MHP in Blood Transfusion, handling analyser downtime in Biochemistry, or processing urgent results in Microbiology, my focus remains on patient safety, accuracy, and professionalism, even under pressure.

Question 113:

Can you tell us an example of when you delivered a high standard of service and what was the impact on the recipient?

Background:

Delivering a high standard of service in a biomedical laboratory means ensuring that patient results are accurate, reliable, and timely. It reflects professionalism, competence, and adherence to laboratory quality systems such as ISO 15189. High standards are achieved by following SOPs, maintaining effective communication with clinical teams, and demonstrating accountability in one's work. This question tests your ability to recognise the value of your contribution to patient care and how your actions impact the wider healthcare service.

Points to Consider:

- Definition of high standard of service in the lab context.
- Use examples where applicable to show impact on patients or clinical teams.
- Link to quality, teamwork, and patient outcomes.
- Reflection on what you did and what you learnt.

Answer:

Delivering a high standard of service means ensuring that every result I produce or validate contributes to safe and effective patient care. It involves being thorough, accurate, and responsive while adhering to the laboratory's quality management system and professional standards.

For example, **in Blood Transfusion**, there was a case where a patient required an urgent blood transfusion for a massive haemorrhage. I received the call from the ward, confirmed the patient details carefully, and immediately activated the Massive Haemorrhage Protocol (MHP). I prioritised the sample, performed the group and crossmatch efficiently, and double-checked the compatibility results before issuing the units. At the same time, I communicated regularly with the ward and the biomedical scientist in charge. The blood units were issued within minutes, and the patient stabilised shortly afterwards.

This demonstrated not only technical competence but also calmness and effective communication under pressure, both of which are essential for a high standard of service.

In another instance, while working **in Biochemistry**, an urgent request for electrolytes and renal function tests arrived from A&E for a critically ill patient. I noticed the potassium result was extremely high, which could have been life-threatening. Before releasing it, I verified the result by checking pre-analytical factors that could influence the results like contamination, haemolysis, time of sample collection, and patient's clinical notes. As the pre-analytical checks showed no indication of interference, I repeated the analysis on a different analyser to confirm the accuracy of the result. I then promptly phoned through and released the result to the requesting clinician. The doctor later confirmed that the immediate treatment given based on this result helped to stabilise the patient.

These examples show how a combination of technical accuracy, prioritisation, and effective communication can make a direct positive impact on patient outcomes.

Summary:

Delivering a high standard of service means combining technical accuracy, professional accountability, and effective communication to ensure patient safety. My experiences such as managing urgent transfusion requests in Blood Transfusion and verifying critical results in Biochemistry have shown me how maintaining high standards directly affects patient care and outcomes. By being attentive to detail, following SOPs, and communicating effectively with clinical teams, I ensure that the service I deliver consistently supports patient safety and the overall reputation of the laboratory.

Question 114:

Tell us your difficult decision you had to make recently and how you went about that the decision making, it doesn't have to be lab work?

Background:

In any professional setting, especially in healthcare, making decisions is vital and sometimes difficult ones is part of daily responsibilities. Decision-making reflects judgement, accountability, and emotional intelligence. Whether it's about prioritising patient samples, resolving a conflict, or balancing workload pressures, the ability to make sound, ethical, and evidence-based decisions demonstrates professional maturity. This question assesses how you approach complex situations, the reasoning process you use, and how you balance personal and professional values when making a decision.

Points to Consider:

- Understanding what makes a decision difficult (e.g., ethical, time-critical, or emotionally challenging).
- Steps in decision-making - gathering facts, evaluating options, consulting others, and making a reasoned choice.
- Demonstrating accountability and reflection on the outcome.
- Use examples both in and outside the lab to support your answer.

Answer:

One difficult decision I had to make recently was while working in the Biochemistry section. During a busy out-of-hours shift, I noticed that one of the analysers had started giving inconsistent results for troponin tests, which is a critical cardiac marker. Several A&E samples were already pending, and the second analyser was undergoing maintenance. The decision was whether to continue using the faulty analyser to avoid delay or to temporarily stop testing and switch to the backup manual method, which would take longer but guarantee result accuracy.

I immediately assessed the situation by running quality controls and comparing recent patient results. The discrepancies confirmed that the analyser was unreliable. I informed the duty senior biomedical scientist and made the decision to stop using that analyser. I then processed the urgent samples using the manual method while documenting the incident for engineering follow-up. Although this created a short delay, it prevented the release of incorrect results that could have led to inappropriate clinical decisions for cardiac patients.

That decision reinforced the importance of prioritising patient safety over turnaround time, even when the pressure to deliver quickly is high.

Outside the laboratory, a personal example involved deciding whether to continue a part-time postgraduate course while working full-time. Balancing academic deadlines with laboratory shifts was becoming stressful. After evaluating my workload, financial commitments, and long-term goals, I decided to defer one module. I discussed this with my academic tutor and employer to ensure transparency. That decision helped me maintain both my mental wellbeing and work performance. Reflecting on my action taught me that self-care and time management are key components of professional decision-making.

Summary:

Making difficult decisions requires balancing risks, consulting the right people, and focusing on long-term outcomes rather than immediate convenience. In the laboratory, I prioritise patient safety, compliance, and quality when faced with technical or ethical dilemmas. Outside work, I apply the same reasoning such as gathering facts, seeking advice, and reflecting on what supports sustainable, effective outcomes. Both experiences show that sound decision-making is about responsibility, integrity, and reflection, qualities I bring to every professional situation.

Question 115:

Tell us how you will go about dealing with an analytical error such as out-of-range quality control.

Background:

Analytical errors, such as out-of-range quality control (QC), are part of daily laboratory work and must be handled promptly and systematically to maintain the reliability and accuracy of patient results. Quality Control ensures that analysers, reagents, and methods are performing within acceptable limits as defined by the manufacturer, SOPs, and accreditation standards like ISO 15189. This question tests your understanding of the analytical phase of testing, your problem-solving ability, and how you ensure patient results are not compromised when QC issues arise.

Points to Consider:

- Immediate action when QC is out of range - stop releasing patient results.
- Systematic troubleshooting - check reagents, analyser performance, calibration, and QC materials.
- Consultation and escalation - involve a senior or manager when necessary.
- Documentation and corrective actions - record in the quality log and LIMS where applicable.
- Revalidation - ensure QC is back in range before resuming testing.
- Use practical examples to support your answer.

Answer:

When I encounter an out-of-range QC result, my first step is to stop reporting patient results from that analyser or batch. I then quarantine any affected patient samples until the issue is resolved.

Next, I begin a systematic troubleshooting process following the SOP:

- Re-run the QC sample to rule out a random error, such as a pipetting, not properly mixed, underfilled or loading issue.

- If it remains out of range, I check the expiry date, lot number, and integrity of the QC material and reagents - ensuring they have been stored correctly, not contaminated etc.

- I review the calibration status of the analyser. If it has been some time since the last calibration or a recent reagent or lot change, I would recalibrate.

- I also check the maintenance log - issues such as blocked probes, temperature fluctuations, or reagent contamination can all cause QC failure.

If these steps do not correct the issue, I would escalate to a senior biomedical scientist or section manager for further investigation, possibly contacting the engineer or manufacturer if instrument fault is suspected.

Once corrective action has been implemented, I re-run the QC until it falls back within the acceptable range, documenting all actions taken in the quality control log, maintenance log, and non-conformance record. Only then do I resume testing and release patient results.

Example 1 - Biochemistry:

During a shift, the ALT QC result was persistently out of range. I checked and found that a new batch of reagent had been loaded. I verified the calibration curve, recalibrated the analyser, and re-ran QC, which then returned to range. I documented the event in Q-Pulse and notified the senior BMS for follow-up with the supplier.

Example 2 - Haematology:

I once encountered an abnormal white cell QC on a Sysmex analyser. After verifying that reagents were fine, I found a clot in the sample probe. Following cleaning and daily maintenance, QC values returned to range. This confirmed a mechanical rather than a reagent issue.

Example 3 - Blood Transfusion:

While performing daily QC on antibody screening cells, one of the screening cells failed. I immediately replaced the QC cell with a fresh one from a new batch, repeated testing, and logged the batch failure. The incident was also reported to the senior BMS and supplier, ensuring traceability and continuous quality assurance.

Summary:

Dealing with an analytical error such as out-of-range QC requires a systematic, calm, and evidence-based approach. The key is to stop reporting patient results, investigate the cause following the SOP, document every step, and ensure corrective action is verified before resuming testing. This process protects patient safety, maintains laboratory integrity, and demonstrates adherence to ISO 15189

standards and the principles of continual quality improvement.

Question 116:

What would you do if the analyser is functioning correctly, but the control result is still out of range?

Background:

In the laboratory, internal quality control (IQC) is an essential part of ensuring reliable patient results. Even if an analyser appears to be functioning normally, out-of-range control results indicate potential analytical or pre-analytical issues that must be investigated before releasing any patient results. ISO 15189 and SOPs require that all quality control failures be resolved and documented before patient testing can continue. This question tests your understanding of troubleshooting processes, quality assurance, and safe laboratory practice.

Points to Consider:

- Understanding of IQC and its role in ensuring analytical accuracy.
- Stepwise approach to troubleshooting an out-of-range control.
- Importance of not releasing patient results until the issue is resolved.
- Escalation process if issue persists.
- Documentation of non-conformance and corrective action.
- Use of practical examples where appropriate to support your answer (biochemistry, haematology, blood transfusion).

Answer:

If the analyser is functioning correctly but the control result is still out of range, I would not proceed with patient testing until the issue is fully resolved, and controls are back within acceptable limits. Out-of-range QC results, even with a functioning analyser, may point to issues such as deteriorated reagents, expired controls, pipetting errors, or storage temperature deviations.

My approach would follow a structured troubleshooting process:

- **Check the control material** - I would first confirm the control's integrity by checking the expiry date, storage conditions, and whether it has been prepared and mixed properly. For example, **in Biochemistry**, if the serum control was left out of the fridge too long, it may give erroneous results even if the analyser is fine.

- **Repeat the control** - I would re-run the same control. If the result is still out of range, I would open a new vial of control material to eliminate the possibility of control degradation.

- **Check reagents and calibrations** - Next, I would review reagent expiry dates, calibration validity, and lot numbers. **In Haematology**, for example, an out-of-range control might occur if calibration is outdated or if reagent carryover has occurred.

- **Perform maintenance or background checks** - Even though the analyser appears fine, I would still check probe cleanliness, tubing, and temperature stability, as small blockages or evaporation issues can cause subtle errors.

- **Use a secondary analyser or peer comparison** - If available, I would run the same control on a different analyser to compare results. For example, **in Biochemistry**, comparing control results across two analysers can help identify whether the issue is analyser- or reagent-related.

- **Escalate the issue** - If all checks are satisfactory but the control remains out of range, I would escalate to the senior biomedical scientist or duty manager for further investigation. It may also be necessary to contact the manufacturer's technical support for additional troubleshooting.

- **Document and investigate** - Finally, I would document the incident as a non-conformance in the laboratory's QMS (e.g., Q-Pulse) and record all corrective actions taken. Patient results during this period would be withheld until the control is within the acceptable range again.

Practical Example:

In a biochemistry laboratory, I once encountered a situation where the analyser's daily checks were fine, but both normal and abnormal controls for urea and creatinine were out of range. After confirming that reagents and analyser performance were stable, I checked the control lot number and discovered that the control vial had been stored outside the recommended 2–8°C range overnight. I immediately opened a fresh control vial and repeated the IQC, which resolved the issue and returned the results to within range. I then logged the incident as a non-conformance and reminded the team about the correct storage of controls.

Summary:

When control results are out of range despite the analyser functioning properly, it is vital to stop patient testing and conduct systematic troubleshooting. This includes verifying control integrity, reagents, and calibration, re-running controls, comparing across analysers, and escalating when necessary. Every step must be documented in line with ISO 15189 and SOPs. This careful, structured approach ensures that patient safety is protected, analytical accuracy is maintained, and continuous quality improvement is achieved within the laboratory.

Question 117:

What do you understand about QMS and what it means to the laboratory?

Background:

Quality Management System (QMS) is an essential framework that ensures the accuracy, reliability, and consistency of laboratory results. It forms the foundation for compliance with ISO 15189 standards, UKAS accreditation, and other regulatory requirements such as MHRA or HTA depending on the department. This question tests your understanding of what a QMS is, how it applies in a pathology setting, and how it helps maintain patient safety and service quality.

Points to Consider:

- Define QMS in your own words.
- Link it to ISO 15189 and UKAS accreditation.
- Explain its impact on quality, consistency, and patient safety.
- Mention QMS tools (e.g., document control, non-conformance logs, audit, EQA/IQC, training records).
- Provide examples where appropriate to support your answer.
- Show how QMS promotes continuous improvement and accountability.

Answer:

A Quality Management System (QMS) is a structured framework that outlines all the processes, procedures, and responsibilities required to achieve and maintain consistent quality in laboratory services. It ensures that every stage of laboratory work from sample receipt to result reporting is carried out to the highest possible standard in line with ISO 15189 and regulatory guidelines.

In practical terms, QMS means that the laboratory has an organised system for document control, staff training, equipment maintenance, risk management, audit, incident reporting, and continuous improvement.

For example, **in Haematology,** the QMS ensures that all analysers are calibrated and maintained as per schedule, that IQC and EQA are regularly monitored, and that any analytical or clerical errors are documented and investigated through the non-conformance process. Similarly, **in Blood Transfusion**, adherence to MHRA and BSH guidelines through the QMS ensures traceability, product safety, and compliance with national standards.

When a non-conformance occurs such as an out-of-range quality control or sample labelling issue, it is logged in the QMS (for example, Q-Pulse). This triggers an investigation, root cause analysis, and implementation of corrective and preventive actions (CAPA) to ensure the issue does not recur.

The QMS also plays a vital role in staff training and competency. Each member of staff must be trained, assessed, and authorised for specific tasks. For example, new staff are expected to undergo induction, competency assessments, and training or retraining as required. All of this is documented within the QMS to ensure accountability and regulatory compliance.

The system also ensures the laboratory is ready for UKAS inspections, where assessors review evidence of compliance, traceability, and continuous improvement activities.

Practical Example:

In a Biochemistry department, I once identified inconsistencies in the turnaround time for urgent samples. Through QMS-driven audit and data review, we discovered delays were due to manual logging of urgent samples instead of using the automated LIMS flag. Based on the findings, we updated the SOP and retrained staff, which significantly improved turnaround time and reduced errors. This example shows how QMS promotes evidence-based improvements in patient care.

Summary:

A Quality Management System is the backbone of laboratory practice, ensuring that all work is standardised, traceable, and continuously improving. It supports compliance with ISO

15189, maintains accreditation, safeguards patient safety, and fosters a culture of accountability and improvement. In essence, QMS provides the structure and confidence that every result released by the laboratory is accurate, reliable, and produced through validated processes, which is fundamental to delivering high-quality patient care.

Question 118:

What do you understand about External Quality Assurance (EQA)?

Background:

External Quality Assurance (EQA) is one of the most important aspects of maintaining high-quality and reliable laboratory results. It is part of the wider Quality Management System (QMS) and ensures that the laboratory's performance is comparable to others nationally and internationally. This question is designed to assess your understanding of what EQA is, its purpose, and how it contributes to laboratory accuracy, staff competency, and accreditation compliance (e.g., UKAS and ISO 15189).

Points to Consider:

- Define EQA clearly in your own words.
- Explain its purpose - accuracy, consistency, and benchmarking.
- Describe the process - participation, analysis, corrective action.
- Mention its difference from IQC (Internal Quality Control).
- Provide examples where appropriate (Haematology, Biochemistry, Microbiology, Histopathology, Blood Transfusion).
- Highlight its link to QMS, UKAS, and continuous improvement.

Answer:

External Quality Assurance (EQA) is an independent assessment process that allows a laboratory to evaluate the accuracy and reliability of its results by comparing them with those of other laboratories performing the same tests. It serves as an external check to confirm that laboratory results are correct, consistent, and in line with accepted national or international standards.

Typically, EQA samples are distributed by accredited schemes such as UK NEQAS (United Kingdom National External Quality Assessment Service), WEQAS, or QCMD. These samples are processed by the laboratory in the same way as routine patient samples. The results are then submitted to the EQA provider for comparison with peer group data.

If the laboratory's results fall outside the acceptable range, an investigation is carried out to identify the cause, whether due to reagent issues, instrument malfunction, calibration drift, or operator error. Corrective and preventive actions (CAPA) are documented within the QMS, and any required retraining or recalibration is carried out to restore accuracy. For example, **in Haematology,** EQA helps ensure the accuracy of full blood count (FBC) parameters such as haemoglobin or platelet counts across different analysers. **In Biochemistry,** EQA confirms consistency of analytes like creatinine or glucose, which are critical for patient diagnosis and treatment. **In Microbiology,** participation in EQA schemes helps ensure the correct identification and antimicrobial susceptibility of organisms. Similarly, **in Histopathology,** EQA assesses staining quality or diagnostic interpretation consistency among pathologists.

EQA performance is also reviewed regularly during UKAS inspections as evidence of the laboratory's commitment to quality and continuous improvement.

Practical Example:

In Blood Transfusion, I once participated in a UK NEQAS EQA scheme for antibody screening. Our result was initially flagged as "out of consensus." I collaborated with the senior biomedical scientist to investigate the issue. We discovered that the cell panel reagent used was nearing expiry, which affected antigen reactivity. After replacing the reagent and repeating the test, our results returned within the expected range. The incident was recorded in the non-conformance log, and the finding was discussed at the quality meeting to raise staff awareness and prevent recurrence.

Summary:

External Quality Assurance ensures laboratories produce accurate, reliable, and comparable results by providing an independent assessment of performance. It promotes accountability, enhances staff competency, and drives continuous improvement through the QMS. Regular participation in EQA schemes not only supports UKAS and ISO 15189 compliance but also underpins patient safety by ensuring confidence in every laboratory result reported.

Question 119:

What importance do you place on CPD (Continuing Professional Development)?

Background:

Continuing Professional Development (CPD) is a regulatory and professional requirement for Biomedical Scientists and other healthcare professionals. It ensures that practitioners remain competent, current, and confident in their roles. The Health and Care Professions Council (HCPC) requires all registrants to maintain a CPD portfolio demonstrating continuous learning and improvement. This question assesses your understanding of why CPD matters, how it contributes to personal growth, professional competence, and ultimately improves patient care.

Points to Consider:

- Define CPD and its purpose.
- Discuss personal and professional importance of CPD.
- Highlight types of CPD (formal and informal learning).
- Link CPD to HCPC, IBMS, ISO 15189, and QMS requirements.
- Provide examples of CPD activities you have undertaken.
- Emphasise how CPD improves patient safety, service quality, and career progression.

Answer:

Continuing Professional Development (CPD) is a structured approach to learning that helps me continually update and improve my knowledge, skills, and performance as a Biomedical Scientist. It ensures that I remain competent, adaptable, and aligned with current best practices, new technologies, and evolving regulations in the laboratory.

I place great importance on CPD because it not only fulfils the HCPC and IBMS professional requirements but also enhances my ability to deliver safe and effective patient care. For example, by engaging in CPD, I stay informed about changes in UKAS accreditation standards, MHRA blood safety alerts, and new laboratory methodologies.

There are several types of CPD I prioritise:

- **Academic CPD:** Completing formal qualifications or IBMS Specialist Portfolio.

- **Training CPD:** Attending internal and external training such as new analyser training or blood transfusion competency updates.

- **Conference CPD:** Participating in scientific meetings such as IBMS Congress or online webinars to learn about emerging techniques.

- **Reflective CPD:** Documenting learning from incidents, audits, or case reviews to identify areas of improvement.

- **Research and Quality CPD:** Engaging in audits or quality improvement projects that align with QMS principles and ISO 15189 requirements.

For example, after attending a CPD session on traceability in blood transfusion, I helped update our local SOPs to reflect the new MHRA guidelines. Similarly, after completing an EQA interpretation course, I was able to support junior colleagues in understanding how to identify and respond to performance outliers.

Summary:

CPD is essential for maintaining competence, improving service delivery, and ensuring patient safety. I view CPD not as a regulatory obligation but as a professional responsibility and personal investment. Through CPD, I can stay up to date with scientific advancements, adapt to new laboratory challenges, and continue to contribute effectively to team development and quality improvement. In short, CPD sustains both professional excellence and public trust in the work we do as Biomedical Scientists.

Question 120:

We want to let you know you are expected to work shifts day, weekend, bank holidays and night shifts if successful - how do you feel about this?

Background:

Working as a Biomedical Scientist requires flexibility to maintain 24/7 laboratory service delivery. Many diagnostic laboratories operate shift patterns, including days, nights, weekends, and bank holidays, to ensure uninterrupted patient testing and timely results. This question assesses your willingness, adaptability, and understanding of the responsibilities and challenges associated with working across different shifts. It also tests how you balance work-life commitments while maintaining high professional standards and patient safety during both day and night duties.

Points to Consider:

- Show understanding that shift work is essential for patient care.
- Highlight your flexibility and adaptability to different shift patterns.
- Discuss how you maintain focus, performance, and wellbeing during nights.
- Mention teamwork and communication during shift handovers.
- Use examples of experience working shifts or adapting to changing schedules.
- Emphasise commitment to quality and safety, regardless of time of day.

Answer:

I fully understand that working both day and night shifts is an essential part of providing continuous laboratory services, especially in a hospital setting where patient care depends on timely results. I am comfortable with this expectation and view it as an important responsibility that ensures the laboratory continues to support emergency and routine work 24 hours a day.

I have experience working shifts, including nights and weekends, and have developed effective strategies to manage my workload and maintain alertness. For example, during out-of-hours (OOH) shifts, I often work independently, performing urgent biochemistry or haematology tests such as blood gases, crossmatches, and coagulation studies. I ensure all results are validated promptly and any critical results are communicated immediately to clinicians, maintaining both efficiency and accuracy under pressure.

During day shifts, I focus on team-based tasks such as quality control reviews, analyser maintenance, and training junior staff. This combination of collaborative work during the day and independent work at night helps me stay adaptable and confident in all situations.

I also recognise the importance of effective handover between shifts. I always make sure any pending issues such as instrument flags, or ongoing investigations are communicated clearly to the staff member coming to take over from me. That way I ensure service maintenance and continuity. To manage wellbeing, I maintain a consistent sleep routine before and after night shifts, stay hydrated, and take short breaks, when possible, to stay alert and safe.

Summary:

I fully accept and am prepared for working both day and night shifts as part of my professional role. I understand that flexibility is vital to ensuring round the clock patient care and laboratory efficiency. My previous experience and commitment to maintaining high standards, communication, and wellbeing across shifts ensure that I can always contribute effectively and reliably to the laboratory service.

Question 121:

What laboratory analysers do you use?

Background:

Biomedical Scientists work with a range of analysers depending on their laboratory discipline such as Haematology, Blood Transfusion, Biochemistry, Microbiology, or Histopathology. This question assesses your practical experience, technical competence, and familiarity with modern laboratory instrumentation and automation systems. It also evaluates your ability to operate, maintain, and troubleshoot analysers in accordance with the manufacturer's guidelines, ISO 15189 standards, and local SOPs.

Points to Consider:

- Mention analysers you have direct experience operating (e.g., Abbott, Sysmex, Siemens, Roche, etc.).
- Include discipline-specific examples (Haematology, Biochemistry, Blood Transfusion, Microbiology, Histopathology).
- Briefly describe key tasks operation, calibration, maintenance, troubleshooting, and quality control.
- Demonstrate understanding of data management systems (LIMS, middleware).
- Link to accuracy, reliability, and patient safety.

Answer:

I have worked with a range of analysers across different pathology departments, which has strengthened my technical and analytical skills.

In Haematology, I have used the Sysmex XN series, DXH 800 Beckman coulter for full blood counts and reticulocyte analysis. I routinely performed daily maintenance, calibration, and internal quality control checks, ensuring results were within acceptable limits before releasing them. I am also familiar with the Stago STA Compact Max, Werfen Top 550, Sysmex CS-2000i analyser for coagulation testing, where I regularly verified results and reviewed abnormal flags before validation.

In Biochemistry, I have worked with Roche Cobas 8000 series and Abbott Alinity platforms. My responsibilities included performing daily and weekly maintenance, running IQCs, reviewing Levy-Jennings charts for QC performance, and troubleshooting analyser errors or reagent issues. I also participated in verification of new reagent lots, ensuring correlation with existing batches according to SOP and ISO15189 requirements.

In Blood Transfusion, I have experience using the Bio-Rad IH-1000 and Ortho Vision for antibody screening, crossmatching, and blood grouping. I ensure all results match LIMS records and that patient identification and sample integrity are checked at every stage. I am confident in performing analyser maintenance, temperature monitoring of reagent fridges and incubators, and participating in IQC and EQA programmes.

In Microbiology, I have used the BD Phoenix M50 for microbial identification and antibiotic susceptibility testing, the Vitek 2 Compact for automated organism identification, and the BD BACTEC FX for blood culture detection. I ensure all instruments are monitored for incubation times, contamination alerts, and temperature controls, while also reviewing results alongside Gram stain findings for correlation.

In Histopathology, I have experience using the Leica ASP300 tissue processor for specimen processing, the Leica RM2235 microtome for sectioning, and the Ventana BenchMark Ultra for automated immunohistochemistry staining. I also worked with the Hologic ThinPrep system for cytology sample preparation. I ensured all equipment was maintained according to schedule, with daily start-up checks and reagent quality verification.

Additionally, I am comfortable using Laboratory Information Management Systems (LIMS) such as WinPath, Telepath, and Clinisys, and middleware systems like Instrument Manager, which support result verification and analyser connectivity.

Summary:

I have hands-on experience with a range of laboratory analysers across Haematology, Biochemistry, Blood Transfusion, Microbiology. I am competent in operating, maintaining, and troubleshooting analysers such as Sysmex XN Line 9000, Roche Cobas, IH-500, and Vitek in line with ISO15189 and SOP standards. My ability to integrate analyser performance with quality control processes and LIMS reporting ensures accurate, timely, and reliable results that directly support patient diagnosis and management.

Question 122:

How many samples do you work on daily?

Background:

The number of samples processed daily in a laboratory depends on the department, workload, staffing levels, and shift pattern. This question assesses your understanding of workload management, attention to detail under pressure, and your ability to maintain accuracy and quality when handling high sample volumes. It also evaluates your awareness of how automation, teamwork, and time management contribute to an efficient laboratory workflow. **Points to Consider:**

- Acknowledge that sample volume varies by department and shift (day, evening, or night).
- Mention how you manage high workloads while maintaining accuracy and TAT.
- Discuss teamwork, organisation, and use of automation to handle volume efficiently.
- Use practical examples to support your answer.
- Link your approach to quality, patient safety, and ISO15189 compliance.

Answer:

The number of samples I work on daily depends on the department and shift pattern. However, regardless of volume, I always prioritise accuracy, quality, and turnaround time.

In Haematology, during busy day shifts, I typically process between 400 - 600 full blood count and 300 – 500 coagulation samples per day using analysers like the Sysmex XN series and Stago STA Compact Max. I manage this workload by batching samples efficiently, performing analyser maintenance early in the shift, and continuously monitoring QC results to ensure accuracy before releasing patient results.

In Biochemistry, I often handle 500 - 800 samples per day, depending on hospital size and service demand. Working on platforms such as the Roche Cobas 8000 or Abbott Alinity c, I ensure urgent (STAT) samples are prioritised using LIMS flagging, while maintaining a steady flow of routine work. I also check for analyser flags or delta failures before validation to ensure patient results are accurate.

In Blood Transfusion, while sample numbers are usually lower. I usually process between 50 - 100 group and save and additional 10 – 15 crossmatch per day. This is outside issuing blood components and products following already processed samples or patient's history. I ensure every group, screen, and crossmatch is handled with full traceability, following SOPs and double-checking units before issue, particularly during high-demand scenarios such as Major Haemorrhage Protocols (MHPs).

In Microbiology, daily workloads can be large depending on the sample type. For example, I have processed around 150 - 200 samples for culture and sensitivity using BD BACTEC and Vitek 2 systems. I ensure timely sub-culturing, accurate inoculation, and daily review of growth reports to avoid backlogs.

In Histopathology, depending on the workload, I may handle 80 - 150 specimens daily. This includes embedding, sectioning, staining (manual or automated), and preparing slides for pathologist review. I maintain attention to detail, especially when matching cassettes and slides to patient details, as errors at this stage can significantly impact diagnosis.

Overall, regardless of the department, I manage high sample volumes through effective teamwork, strong time management, and strict adherence to SOPs. I ensure that every result released meets the laboratory's quality and safety standards in line with ISO 15189.

Summary:

The number of samples I process daily varies depending on the department. For example, high volumes in Haematology (500 – 600) and Biochemistry (700 – 800), moderate in Microbiology (200 – 400), and lower but highly detailed work

in Blood Transfusion and Histopathology (50 – 150). Regardless of workload, I maintain quality, accuracy, and turnaround times by staying organised, working collaboratively, and following SOPs. This ensures that all results are accurate, traceable, and contribute to effective patient care.

Question 123:

How do you validate your results?

Background:

Result validation is an essential part of laboratory quality management and patient safety. It ensures that only accurate, reliable, and clinically meaningful results are released. Biomedical Scientists must validate results by assessing quality control (QC), analyser performance, sample integrity, delta checks, and clinical correlation before authorising results. This question tests your understanding of both analytical and post-analytical validation, as well as how you respond to abnormal or unexpected results.

Points to Consider:

- Understanding the difference between technical and clinical validation.
- Checking sample integrity before validating results (e.g. clotted, haemolysed, lipaemic, or insufficient samples).
- Reviewing QC data, analyser flags, and delta checks.
- Ensuring correlation with patient history or previous results.
- Repeating tests or escalating where necessary.
- Using SOPs, manufacturer guidance, and clinical knowledge.
- Provide examples to support your answer where appropriate (Haematology, Biochemistry, Blood Transfusion, Microbiology, Histopathology).

Answer:

Result validation involves a structured and evidence-based approach to ensure reliability before authorisation. I begin by considering pre-analytical factors that could affect accuracy such as clotted or insufficient samples in Haematology, haemolysed or lipaemic samples in Biochemistry, or contaminated samples in Microbiology. These issues can compromise results, so I ensure that the sample integrity is suitable before proceeding or validating.

Once the sample is deemed suitable, I move to technical validation by confirming that internal quality control (IQC) results are within acceptable ranges and that the analyser is functioning correctly with no outstanding flags. For example, **in Haematology**, I check the Sysmex XN for any abnormal flags (e.g. platelet clumps, blasts, atypical lymphocytes) and review the blood film if necessary. I also perform delta checks to compare the result with previous data. For example, MCV delta check fail. So, any large or unexplained variation prompts further investigation or a repeat test.

In Biochemistry, if a result appears abnormal (e.g. a high potassium), I assess whether the sample was haemolysed, lipaemic, or diluted. I also verify the analyser flag and review the patient's clinical history. If results remain inconsistent after reanalysis, I consult a senior BMS before releasing or requesting a repeat sample.

In Blood Transfusion, I validate by ensuring all patient identifiers match perfectly, confirming that the antibody screen, crossmatch, and unit selection align. If a discrepancy arises, such as an unexpected antibody pattern, I investigate before any issue or authorisation.

In Microbiology, I confirm the consistency of growth patterns, gram stains, and susceptibility profiles. For example, if an organism shows an unexpected resistance pattern, I confirm its identity with MALDI-TOF or Vitek 2 and verify susceptibility manually if required. This allows me to decide whether to validate result the result immediately or request advice from senior BMS, consultant, or ask for sample repeat.

In Histopathology, validation involves ensuring that the slide labels, tissue blocks, and reports match the correct patient, and that all controls and stains have been appropriately interpreted before sign-out by the pathologist.

If any irregularities are detected during validation, I follow SOPs for corrective action, which may include repeat testing, checking reagents, recalibrating instruments, or escalating to a senior colleague. Also, ensure that every step is documented for traceability.

Summary:

Before validating results, I assess the sample quality, review QC performance and analyser status, consider pre-analytical factors such as haemolysis, lipaemia, or clots, and perform clinical correlation with patient history and previous data. Across all departments, I apply SOPs, professional judgement, and good communication to ensure that only accurate, traceable, and clinically valid results are released. This process maintains the laboratory's quality standards and ensures safe, effective patient care.

Question 124:

What quality management processes are carried out in your lab and how have you been a part of it?

Background:

Quality Management Systems (QMS) are the foundation of laboratory practice, ensuring accuracy, consistency, and compliance with accreditation standards such as UKAS ISO 15189 and regulatory bodies like MHRA or HTA. Biomedical Scientists play a key role in maintaining quality by participating in internal and external audits, non-conformance investigations, document control, training, risk assessment, and continuous improvement. This question tests your understanding of how QMS principles are practically applied in daily laboratory work and how you personally contribute to quality assurance, safety, and compliance.

Points to Consider:

- Define QMS and its importance in laboratory governance.
- Mention specific quality processes in your department (IQC, EQA, audits, document review, incident reporting, training records, etc.).
- Describe your personal involvement in maintaining or improving quality.
- Provide examples to support your answer where applicable (e.g., Blood Transfusion, Biochemistry, Microbiology, Histopathology).
- Emphasise the link between quality processes, accreditation, and patient safety.

Answer:

Quality management processes are integral to the functioning of any accredited laboratory. In my current and previous roles, I have actively contributed to several QMS activities designed to uphold compliance with UKAS ISO 15189 and maintain high analytical and professional standards.

In Haematology and Blood Transfusion, I routinely participate in internal quality control (IQC) checks before processing patient samples and review external quality assurance (EQA) results to ensure our performance is within acceptable limits. When EQA results deviate, I help investigate the root cause and document corrective and preventive actions (CAPA) on the Q-Pulse system. I also take part in daily equipment maintenance, calibration verification, and temperature monitoring to ensure all instruments are performing optimally.

In Biochemistry, I contribute to quality management by performing and reviewing Levey-Jennings charts, verifying QC trends, and escalating when systematic errors are detected. I have participated in a local audit that assessed sample turnaround time and non-conformances, which led to recommendations that improved workflow efficiency.

In Microbiology, I assist in media QC, checking for contamination or growth suitability, and ensure that susceptibility testing adheres to EUCAST standards. Similarly, **in Histopathology,** I help maintain embedding and staining quality checks, ensuring control slides stain appropriately before patient slides are validated.

I have also participated in document control by reviewing and updating standard operating procedures (SOPs) to reflect current practice and ensure staff compliance. Additionally, I have logged and investigated non-conformances. For example, analyser downtime and sample mislabelling to identify underlying causes and prevent recurrence.

My involvement in training and competency assessments of junior staff is also part of maintaining quality, ensuring that everyone working in the lab meets the required competence standards.

Summary:

I actively contribute to several quality management processes, including IQC, EQA, audits, non-conformance management, SOP review, training, and equipment maintenance. By following QMS procedures, I help ensure continuous improvement, maintain UKAS and MHRA compliance, and safeguard patient results. Quality management is not just a system to me, it is part of daily professional practice that underpins accuracy, safety, and patient confidence in laboratory services.

Question 125:

Take me through the trainings you have been involved in.

Background:

Training in a pathology laboratory is vital to maintain staff competence, ensure patient safety, and support continuous professional development (CPD). Biomedical scientists are expected to engage in formal and informal training, including on-the-job mentorship, competency assessments, workshops, and external courses. This question tests your understanding of training principles, your involvement in staff development, and how training contributes to quality service delivery.

Points to Consider:

- Different types of training: induction, competency-based, refresher, technical workshops, CPD courses, conferences.
- Your role: trainer, trainee, or both.
- How training impacts competence, patient safety, and laboratory standards.
- Give examples to support your answer (Biochemistry, Haematology, Microbiology, Histopathology).

Answer:

Throughout my career as a Biomedical Scientist, I have been actively involved in various forms of training, both as a learner and as a trainer. When I joined new laboratories, I completed induction training, which included familiarisation with SOPs, laboratory safety procedures, LIMS, and departmental workflows. This ensured I could perform my duties competently and safely from the outset.

In my current role, I have participated in competency-based training for new instruments and analysers. For example, **in Biochemistry,** I was trained on a new automated analyser, where I learned calibration, maintenance, and quality control procedures, ensuring compliance with ISO 15189. Similarly, **in Microbiology**, I underwent training on antimicrobial susceptibility testing according to EUCAST standards, and **in Histopathology**, I participated in workshops on tissue processing and staining techniques.

I have also been involved in training junior staff and Band 5 scientists, using a structured approach that combines demonstration, supervised practice, and competency assessment. For example, I mentored a newly qualified Band 5 in Haematology, guiding them through full blood count sample processing, analyser validation, and result verification. I provided feedback, corrected mistakes, and ensured they were confident before signing off their competency.

Additionally, I have attended CPD workshops and conferences, which have enhanced my knowledge in areas such as transfusion medicine, quality management, and laboratory safety. These training opportunities have enabled me to share best practices with colleagues, implement improvements within the laboratory, and meet the requirements for professional registration.

Summary:

I have been involved in a variety of training activities, including induction, competency-based learning, mentorship, and CPD courses across Biochemistry, Haematology, Microbiology, and Histopathology. My participation has helped me maintain competence, support colleague's development, and ensure the delivery of safe and high-quality patient results. Training is not just about personal growth. It ensures the laboratory functions efficiently and maintains compliance with professional and regulatory standards.

Question 126:

Who do you think our customers are?

Background:

In a pathology laboratory, understanding who the "customers" are is crucial because the service is built around supporting patient care. Customers are not only the patients themselves but also healthcare professionals who rely on laboratory results to make diagnostic and treatment decisions. This question tests your understanding of the laboratory's role in the healthcare ecosystem and the importance of meeting customer needs while maintaining quality and patient safety.

Points to Consider:

- Identify primary and secondary customers (patients, doctors, nurses, other hospital staff).
- Consider external customers (GP surgeries, other Trust hospitals, research organisations).
- Highlight the impact of laboratory service quality on these customers.
- Give practical examples of how you interact with customers or support them.

Answer:

In my view, the customers of a pathology laboratory are both direct and indirect. The primary customers are patients, who rely on accurate and timely results for their diagnosis, treatment, and overall wellbeing. For example, if a critical potassium result is reported quickly and accurately, it can prevent serious complications for the patient.

Secondary customers include clinicians, nurses, and other healthcare professionals who rely on the laboratory to provide accurate results for informed decision-making. For example, a doctor reviewing blood culture results in Microbiology or a nurse checking a haemoglobin result in Haematology depends on the laboratory to deliver timely and reliable information.

There are also external customers, such as GP surgeries, other Trust hospitals, or research organisations that may send samples to the lab. Maintaining good communication, quick turnaround times, and adherence to SOPs ensures we meet their expectations.

Summary:

Laboratory customers include patients, clinicians, nurses, other healthcare professionals, and external organisations. By providing accurate, timely, and reliable results, the laboratory directly supports patient care and helps healthcare staff make informed decisions. My role is to ensure every result delivered meets these customer expectations while

maintaining quality and safety standards, whether in Biochemistry, Haematology, Microbiology, or Histopathology.

Question 127:

Do you understand how the NHS system is structured and how it differs from where you previously worked?

Background:

The National Health Service (NHS) is the UK's public healthcare system, founded on the principles of providing safe, high-quality care to all patients, free at the point of use. For professionals joining from international or private laboratories, understanding the NHS structure and governance is essential. The NHS places strong emphasis on quality management, documentation, and accountability to ensure consistency and patient safety across the UK. This question assesses your understanding of the NHS framework and how it compares to your previous work environment.

Points to Consider:

- Structure of NHS: Primary, Secondary, and Tertiary care.
- Quality governance and regulatory bodies (UKAS, MHRA, HTA, HCPC, NHS England).
- Key differences between NHS and international/private laboratory systems.
- Adaptability and commitment to NHS values and continuous improvement.
- Practical examples showing understanding and readiness to integrate.

Answer:

Yes, I understand that the NHS is the UK's publicly funded healthcare system, organised into primary care (such as general practitioners and community services), secondary care (hospitals and diagnostic laboratories), and tertiary care (specialised centres like regional reference labs or transplant units).

Within this structure, every NHS laboratory operates under a strong quality management system (QMS) that ensures accurate, timely, and safe results for patients. The NHS is regulated by key external bodies such as:

- UKAS, which accredits laboratories to ISO 15189 standards.
- MHRA, which ensures safe use of reagents, blood components, and medical devices.
- HTA, which governs tissue handling and storage.
- HCPC, which regulates Biomedical Scientists' professional conduct and registration.

In my previous hospital laboratory overseas, while we also emphasised quality and patient care, the system was often less formalised. For example, internal quality control (IQC) was done routinely, but participation in external quality assurance (EQA) schemes such as UK NEQAS was limited or not nationally standardised. Documentation and incident reporting were often paper-based rather than through a digital system like Q-Pulse or LIMS-linked error tracking used in the NHS.

Since working and training in an NHS laboratory, I have adapted to its structured systems. For example, during equipment verification in Biochemistry, we followed a strict protocol involving method validation, performance verification, and measurement of uncertainty prior to clinical use, all fully in line with ISO 15189 requirements. This level of regulation ensures consistency across NHS Trusts and minimises risk to patients.

I have also learned the importance of multidisciplinary teamwork within the NHS. For example, during a Massive Haemorrhage Protocol (MHP) in Blood Transfusion, effective communication between Biomedical Scientists, clinicians, and porters ensured blood products were issued rapidly and safely. This type of structured coordination reflects the NHS's patient-centred focus and collaborative culture, which may not always be present in smaller or less integrated healthcare systems abroad.

Summary:

The NHS differs from international healthcare systems mainly in its structured organisation, national quality governance, and emphasis on patient safety. Every laboratory process is guided by SOPs, accreditation standards, and professional accountability. Having previously worked in a fast-paced hospital overseas, I bring valuable experience in adaptability, resource management, and commitment to continuous improvement. These skills align well with NHS values of care, respect, and quality. Working within the NHS allows me to apply my experience in a more structured environment where patient safety and quality are central to every decision.

Question 128:

What trainings do you think you will need?

Background:

When starting a new role, especially in a different laboratory or Trust, it is important to identify what training will be needed to perform effectively and safely. This question assesses your awareness of professional development needs, understanding of laboratory-specific processes, and willingness to learn. Biomedical Scientists are expected to maintain competence through induction, refresher, and specialist training to ensure compliance with SOPs, quality standards, and patient safety.

Points to Consider:

- Awareness of Trust-specific or departmental induction training.
- Equipment and analyser-specific training.
- QMS, Health and Safety, and IT systems (LIMS, Q-Pulse).
- Specialist and CPD-related training.

- Commitment to continuous professional development and competency assessment.

Answer:

In starting a new role, I believe it is essential to undergo both Trust-wide and department-specific training to ensure safe and effective practice.

Initially, I would expect to complete mandatory induction training, which covers areas such as health and safety, fire safety, infection control, information governance, and patient confidentiality. This helps ensure I understand the policies, procedures, and values specific to the Trust.

From a laboratory perspective, I would require equipment and analyser-specific training, since different hospitals may use different models or suppliers. For example, **in Biochemistry**, I may need hands-on training on analysers such as Abbott Alinity, Roche Cobas, or Siemens Atellica. **In Haematology**, training might cover Sysmex analysers and coagulation systems like IL ACL TOP. Likewise, **in Blood Transfusion,** training may include using ECHO or Ortho Vision analysers and verifying results using the LIMS system.

I would also need refresher or update training in Quality Management Systems (QMS), including document control, incident reporting, non-conformance handling, and internal audits, particularly through platforms such as Q-Pulse.

In addition, I would expect to complete competency-based training to confirm that I can work independently once signed off. This would involve supervised sessions, assessment of work accuracy, and adherence to SOPs and ISO 15189 requirements.

Finally, I would pursue continuing professional development (CPD) opportunities, such as attending internal seminars, external courses (e.g., MHRA Blood Compliance training, IBMS webinars), and case review meetings. These not only build technical skills but also maintain professional registration with the HCPC.

Summary:

The trainings I would need include mandatory Trust induction, analyser and system-specific technical training, QMS and competency assessments, and ongoing CPD to remain current in best practice. I believe in continuous learning and would take every opportunity to update my skills, ensuring that I deliver safe, accurate, and high-quality results in line with Trust and national standards.

Question 129:

How have you helped improve performance in the lab?

Background:

This question assesses your ability to contribute to continuous improvement and quality in laboratory practice. Biomedical Scientists play an active role in enhancing laboratory performance, whether through improving turnaround times, reducing errors, developing procedures, optimising workflow, or mentoring staff. Interviewers want to see evidence of initiative, teamwork, and awareness of quality improvement principles such as audit, root cause analysis, and corrective/preventive actions.

Points to Consider:

- How you identified a problem or performance gap.
- What actions or ideas you introduced to improve the situation.
- Collaboration with others or discussion with management.
- What impact your action had - improved TAT, reduced errors, better teamwork, or enhanced compliance.
- Evidence of learning, audit, or feedback used to drive improvement.

Answer:

Throughout my career, I have always looked for ways to improve laboratory performance by promoting efficiency, accuracy, and teamwork.

In Biochemistry, for example, I noticed that turnaround times were occasionally delayed during peak hours because urgent samples were not being clearly prioritised on the analyser. I proposed a colour-coded tray system and liaised with colleagues to standardise the process across shifts. After implementation, urgent samples were clearly identified and processed faster, improving communication between laboratory and clinical staff.

In Haematology, I contributed to performance improvement by helping review analyser flags and validation criteria. I worked with senior colleagues to update the SOP to ensure consistency across staff members, reducing the number of samples unnecessarily repeated and improving workflow efficiency.

In Blood Transfusion, I participated in a review of near-miss incidents and suggested implementing a double-check log for crossmatch verification. This helped reduce oversight errors and improved traceability. I also contributed to updating competency records to ensure that all staff were current with MHRA and UKAS requirements.

Beyond technical performance, I have also contributed to improvement by mentoring new staff and placement students. For example, I guided trainees in understanding LIMS functions and proper sample workflow, which boosted their confidence and reduced common errors in sample registration and result entry.

Summary:

I believe performance improvement in the lab is a continuous process driven by teamwork, communication, and adherence to quality systems. By identifying workflow issues, suggesting practical solutions, and supporting my colleagues through training and standardisation, I have contributed to more efficient and safer laboratory operations. These

experiences reflect my commitment to maintaining high-quality service delivery and continual improvement in patient care.

Question 130:

A colleague is always proving difficult and not following procedures, what will you do?

Background:

In the laboratory, teamwork and adherence to standard operating procedures (SOPs) are vital for maintaining quality, patient safety, and regulatory compliance. A colleague who is difficult or consistently disregards procedures can pose a risk to workflow, accuracy, and morale. This question tests your understanding of professional communication, conflict resolution, leadership, and quality management, particularly under the principles of duty of candour, accountability, and patient safety.

Points to Consider:

- Stay professional and avoid personal confrontation.
- Address the issue privately and respectfully.
- Emphasise the importance of SOPs for safety and quality.
- Escalate the issue, if necessary, through the proper channels (e.g., senior staff, line manager, quality officer).
- Promote teamwork, mentoring, and positive engagement.
- Document or report incidents in accordance with QMS procedures (e.g., Datix or non-conformance report).

Answer:

If I notice a colleague being difficult or not following laboratory procedures, my first step would be to remain calm and professional. I would avoid confrontation and instead seek to understand the reason behind their behaviour. This is because sometimes non-compliance may be due to misunderstanding, training gaps, or workload stress.

For example, during my time **in Haematology,** I observed a colleague consistently skipping second checks on abnormal results. I approached them privately and explained the importance of verification in maintaining patient safety and compliance with ISO15189. They later admitted feeling pressured by high workload, so we agreed to discuss it with our senior BMS. The team subsequently reviewed the workflow and redistributed the workload, improving compliance and reducing stress for everyone.

If, however, the colleague continued to ignore procedures despite being aware of the correct process, I would escalate the issue to a senior BMS, quality manager, or line manager. This ensures that it is handled formally, in line with departmental policy, while maintaining professionalism and objectivity. In cases where there is a risk to patient safety, I would record the incident in the QMS (for example, through a Datix or non-conformance report) to ensure that appropriate corrective and preventive actions are taken.

In all situations, my aim would be to protect the integrity of the laboratory process and uphold patient safety without an attempt to assign blame, but to encourage improvement and accountability.

Example For Senior or Team Leader Roles:

If I were in a leadership position and noticed a colleague repeatedly being difficult or not following procedures, I would start by handling the matter informally but professionally. I would speak with them privately to understand the underlying cause. This would allow me to determine whether it is due to training gaps, workload pressure, or personal challenges.

For example, **in Clinical Biochemistry**, I once supervised a staff member who frequently bypassed double-checking analyser flags before validating results. In a private discussion, I discovered they were unaware that recent SOP updates had introduced new flagging criteria. I arranged a short refresher training, gave them access to the updated SOP on Q-Pulse, and paired them temporarily with a senior colleague for oversight. This approach corrected the issue quickly and maintained morale.

However, if a colleague continued to disregard procedures despite guidance, I would follow formal escalation routes by reporting the matter to the section manager or quality officer. The incident would also be documented in the QMS (for example, via Datix or a non-conformance report) to ensure traceability and corrective action. Where behaviour posed a potential risk to patient safety, I would prioritise immediate escalation in line with ISO 15189 and the HCPC Code of Conduct.

As a team leader, I would also use this as a learning opportunity for the wider team by organising short discussions or toolbox meetings to reinforce the importance of following SOPs, ensuring everyone feels supported and aware of standards.

Summary:

When dealing with a difficult colleague or non-compliance, I believe in using a calm, professional, and structured approach by addressing issues privately, identifying root causes, and escalating through appropriate channels when necessary. This will helps maintain a safe, high-quality working environment, fosters teamwork, and ensures that patient care is never compromised.

Question 131:

Give an example of a time you had a difficult communication with a clinician.

Background:

In a pathology laboratory, clear communication between biomedical scientists and clinicians is vital to ensure accurate diagnosis, timely patient management, and overall patient safety. However, situations can arise where communication becomes difficult especially in high-pressure circumstances or when clinical staff misunderstand laboratory processes. This question tests your ability to remain professional, communicate effectively, and handle conflict constructively while maintaining patient care standards.

Points to Consider:

- Importance of clear and professional communication between laboratory and clinicians.
- Keeping calm, respectful, and factual under pressure.
- Explaining laboratory processes and limitations in simple terms.
- Using SOPs, policies, and national guidelines to support communication.
- Use examples to support your answer where appropriate: Blood Transfusion, Biochemistry, Microbiology, Histopathology.
- Reflection on lessons learnt.

Answer:

Effective communication is fundamental in laboratory practice, particularly when working with clinicians who rely on laboratory results to make time-critical decisions.

In Blood Transfusion, I once faced a difficult situation when a clinician urgently requested group O negative blood for a patient who already had crossmatched and compatible units available. The doctor insisted that O negative was safer and quicker. I calmly explained that, although O negative is used in emergencies before grouping, in this case, fully crossmatched blood was already available and safer for the patient because it matched their exact blood group, thereby avoiding unnecessary alloimmunisation. I referred to the Trust's transfusion policy and BSH guidelines to support my explanation. By maintaining professionalism and empathy, the situation was resolved, and the correct blood products were issued safely and promptly.

In Biochemistry, I once received a call from a clinician who was upset about a high potassium result that had been rejected and not authorised. The doctor felt the result was urgent and questioned why it was withheld. I explained politely that the sample showed marked haemolysis, which can cause a falsely elevated potassium level. I referred to the LIMS haemolysis index and the laboratory policy, which requires such samples to be rejected to prevent the reporting of inaccurate results. I advised that a repeat sample should be collected using an appropriate phlebotomy technique and reassured the clinician that the request would be prioritised once received. The repeat test returned a normal potassium result, confirming that the initial sample was unsuitable. The clinician appreciated the clear explanation and later acknowledged the importance of good sampling technique. **In Microbiology**, a clinician once became frustrated about the turnaround time for culture and sensitivity results for a septic patient. I explained the microbiological process that cultures require 18–24 hours of incubation for accurate growth identification and advised starting empirical treatment based on the Trust's antimicrobial policy until results were available. Providing context and evidence helped de-escalate the tension and ensured appropriate patient management.

In Histopathology, I encountered a case where a clinician called demanding same-day results for a biopsy that had just been received. I explained that tissue fixation and processing cannot be safely rushed, as poor fixation could compromise diagnostic accuracy. I reassured them that urgent biopsies are always prioritised within the fast-track cancer pathway, and the pathologist would be notified once the slide was ready. This explanation helped the clinician understand that accuracy must never be sacrificed for speed.

Summary:

Difficult communications with clinicians are best managed through professionalism, patience, and evidence-based explanations. I always ensure that I communicate clearly, refer to policies, SOPs, or national guidelines, and focus on maintaining patient safety. These experiences across departments have taught me that clear and respectful dialogue builds mutual trust between laboratory and clinical teams. It also reinforces that even in challenging conversations, maintaining composure and clarity ensures the right decisions are made for patient care.

Question 132:

What would you have done differently now if this occurs?

Background:

Reflective practice is a vital part of continuous improvement in healthcare. It allows Biomedical Scientists to analyse past experiences, learn from them, and apply improved approaches in future situations. This question assesses your ability to reflect constructively, recognise areas for development, and demonstrate professional growth, all of which are key expectations under the HCPC Standards of Proficiency and the ISO 15189 requirements for continual improvement.

Points to Consider:

- Importance of reflection in professional development.
- Identify the situation (link to previous example).
- Explain what was done, what went well, and what could have been improved.
- Highlight what you would do differently now and why.
- Show how reflection has strengthened your future practice.
- Use practical examples to support your answer.

Answer:

Reflecting on the previous situation where I had a difficult communication with a clinician, I've learnt that reflection helps me identify small changes that can improve both communication and laboratory efficiency.

For example, **in the Biochemistry** scenario where a clinician queried a rejected potassium result due to haemolysis, I handled the situation professionally and explained the reason for rejecting the result. However, looking back, what I would do differently now is to ensure proactive communication. For example, by calling the ward as soon as the haemolysed sample was identified, before the clinician contacted the lab. That early communication could have reduced frustration and ensured a repeat sample was sent promptly, minimising delay in patient care.

Similarly, **in Blood Transfusion**, during a major haemorrhage protocol, I realised that while I managed the technical aspects efficiently, I could have communicated more clearly with the clinical team about product availability and turnaround expectations. If faced with a similar situation now, I would ensure regular updates to the clinical team during the process and document all communication on the LIMS or communication log, in line with ISO 15189 documentation standards.

In Microbiology, there was an instance where I explained to a clinician that culture results were pending due to incubation time. Reflecting on that, I would now include information about interim Gram stain results or preliminary findings where available, as this could assist the clinician in making an early, informed decision while waiting for full results.

In Histopathology, after an experience where a clinician was impatient about biopsy turnaround time, I learnt the value of liaising directly with the reporting pathologist to get an accurate estimated reporting time before responding. This ensures I give the clinician realistic expectations backed by accurate information.

Summary:

Reflective learning is one of the cornerstones of laboratory professionalism. In hindsight, I have learnt that early, proactive communication, detailed documentation, and better collaboration with clinical and senior staff can make a significant difference in how issues are managed. If similar situations arise again, I will act more promptly to inform clinicians of issues, provide alternative options when possible, and document every interaction to support transparency and quality assurance. This reflection demonstrates that every challenge, when approached with an open mindset, becomes an opportunity to enhance both professional growth and patient care outcomes.

Question 133:

What do you know about good teamwork?

Background:

Teamwork is one of the key pillars of laboratory practice and patient-centred care. In a multidisciplinary environment like pathology, effective teamwork ensures that results are processed accurately, efficiently, and safely. ISO 15189 and HCPC standards both highlight teamwork as essential for maintaining quality, ensuring continuity of service, and fostering a supportive culture of communication and accountability. This question is testing your understanding of what makes a good team and how collaboration directly impacts laboratory quality and patient outcomes.

Points to Consider:

- Definition of good teamwork.
- Importance of teamwork in the laboratory.
- Elements of effective teamwork (communication, mutual respect, shared responsibility).
- Examples of teamwork where applicable.
- How teamwork improves patient safety, service quality, and staff development.

Answer:

Good teamwork in the laboratory means working collaboratively with colleagues, sharing knowledge, and supporting one another to achieve a common goal, which include delivering accurate, timely, and reliable results for patient care. It is built on clear communication, mutual respect, trust, and shared accountability.

For example, **in Biochemistry,** good teamwork is demonstrated during busy morning shifts when the workload is high. Scientists, medical laboratory assistants, and support staff work together. For example, one may prioritise urgent samples, another performs maintenance or analyser calibration, while another validates results. By sharing responsibilities and communicating clearly, the lab meets turnaround times without compromising quality.

In Haematology, teamwork is especially critical during analyser downtime. When the analyser failed once during a busy afternoon shift, the team divided roles effectively: one scientist contacted the engineer, another manually prepared and processed urgent samples, and a third communicated expected delays to the wards. Because of the strong teamwork and communication, urgent samples were still processed on time, preventing disruption to patient care.

In Blood Transfusion, teamwork plays a vital role during a Major Haemorrhage Protocol (MHP). When the MHP call is activated, one person may prepare the blood packs, another manages LIMS entries, and another double-checks compatibility and product issue. Team coordination ensures that all products are issued quickly, safely, and in accordance with the SOP, which can literally save lives.

In Microbiology, teamwork occurs when managing outbreaks or urgent culture results. For example, if a ward reports a suspected MRSA outbreak, the BMS team and clinical scientists work together to prioritise those samples, communicate results to infection control, and implement follow-up testing.

Similarly, **in Histopathology**, scientists, biomedical support workers, and pathologists collaborate to ensure specimen tracking, tissue processing, and slide preparation are handled efficiently. Everyone's contribution ensures that turnaround targets and diagnostic accuracy are maintained.

Good teamwork also involves providing emotional and professional support to colleagues. This may include helping a colleague who is struggling with their workload, sharing best practice, or offering guidance to new members of staff. It fosters a positive working environment in which individuals feel valued, supported, and motivated to perform at their best.

Summary:

Good teamwork is about collaboration, communication, and mutual accountability to achieve a shared goal, safe and accurate patient results. Whether managing urgent cases in Blood Transfusion, analyser downtime in Biochemistry, or supporting outbreak management in Microbiology, effective teamwork ensures that service quality and patient safety are never compromised. A well-functioning team builds trust, resilience, and consistency, which are essential qualities in a busy laboratory environment. By working together, we strengthen both individual performance and the laboratory's overall contribution to patient care.

Question 134:

What would you do if you have a disagreement with your manager?

Background:

Disagreements in the workplace can occur for many reasons such as differences in opinion, approach, or interpretation of policies or results. The key is not to avoid disagreements but to handle them professionally and constructively. In the laboratory setting, where accuracy, safety, and teamwork are crucial, it is important to resolve issues respectfully to maintain service quality and good working relationships. This question tests your ability to manage conflict, communicate effectively, and demonstrate professionalism.

Points to Consider:

- Stay calm, respectful, and professional.
- Listen and understand the manager's point of view.
- Express your opinion clearly and with evidence or guidelines (SOPs, UKAS, MHRA, ISO 15189, etc.).
- Escalate appropriately if unresolved (e.g., to a senior manager or HR).

- Maintaining patient safety and quality at all times.
- Examples from the lab help show maturity and professionalism.

Answer:

If I ever have a disagreement with my manager, I will approach the situation calmly and respectfully. My first step would be to listen carefully to their point of view to understand their reasoning. Then, I would present my perspective politely, using facts, evidence, and relevant guidelines to support my point.

For example**, in Biochemistry**, if my manager decides to validate a borderline result that I believe requires repeat testing due to haemolysis or sample interference, I will respectfully share my concerns and refer to SOPs or quality procedures. I might say, "According to our policy, results affected by haemolysis should be repeated for accuracy." This keeps the discussion professional and patient focused.

If after discussion we still disagree, I would suggest involving a senior colleague or Quality Lead for further clarification, which is not to challenge authority but to ensure that the final decision aligns with laboratory standards and patient safety.

In Histopathology, for example, if I disagree with the workflow priority for urgent biopsy samples, I will first discuss my concerns directly with my manager. If needed, I could suggest referring to turnaround time standards or national guidelines to find a fair and evidence-based solution.

Similarly, **in Microbiology**, if I feel that an urgent sample should be processed immediately but the manager believes it can wait, I will explain my reasoning (e.g., clinical significance or risk of infection spread). The aim would always be to find common ground, keeping patient care as the top priority.

If the disagreement involved a personal issue or workplace decision (for example, shift allocation or workload distribution), I would still follow the same principle, which is to discuss privately, remain calm, and, if necessary, seek mediation from HR or a senior manager. Maintaining professionalism and mutual respect is key.

Summary:

Disagreements can happen in any workplace, but how they are handled defines professionalism. I believe in open, respectful communication based on facts and guidelines. By listening, explaining my view calmly, and seeking clarification where needed, I ensure that any disagreement is resolved in a constructive way that protects patient safety, service quality, and team harmony. In the end, it's not about being right but it's about ensuring that the best decision is made for the laboratory and patient care.

Question 135:

What would you do if your colleague disagrees with you?

Background:

In any laboratory environment, colleagues may sometimes have different opinions about how to interpret results, prioritise work, or follow certain procedures. This is normal in a multidisciplinary setting where people bring different experiences and training backgrounds. The key is not avoiding disagreement, but knowing how to handle it professionally, respectfully, and constructively. The goal should always be patient safety, teamwork, and service quality.

Points to Consider:

- Stay calm, polite, and professional.
- Listen carefully to your colleague's point of view.
- Refer to objective evidence such as SOPs, QC results, or national guidelines (BSH, MHRA, UKAS, ISO 15189).
- Involve a senior staff or manager if needed for clarification.
- Maintain teamwork and avoid personal conflict.

- Use examples from laboratory practice to support your answer (e.g., Blood Transfusion, Biochemistry, Microbiology, or Histopathology).

Answer:

If a colleague disagrees with me, I will remain calm, professional, and open-minded. I would start by listening carefully to their reasoning and trying to understand their point of view. Sometimes disagreements come from miscommunication or different interpretations of a procedure, and a simple discussion can resolve it.

For example, **in Blood Transfusion**, if a colleague and I disagree about whether a crossmatch is required or an electronic issue is acceptable, I would refer to the laboratory's SOPs or BSH guidelines. I might say, "Let's check the SOP to confirm the policy for this type of request." This approach removes personal opinion and focuses on standard practice to ensure patient safety.

In Biochemistry, if a colleague believes an analyser result should be released but I suspect interference from haemolysis, I will share my concern politely and show how the sample integrity data may have contributed to the type results obtained by referring to the lab SOPs. I would recommend where possible that we review the sample together or consult a senior Biomedical Scientist to make a joint decision. This ensures the right outcome without tension.

In Microbiology, if we disagree about identifying an organism or interpreting an antibiogram, I will suggest reviewing the plate or data together, or if needed, asking for a second opinion from a senior scientist. This encourages learning and avoids unnecessary conflict.

Similarly, **in Histopathology**, if there's a difference in how urgent samples is prioritised, I would discuss it respectfully and agree on a plan that best meets turnaround time targets and clinical urgency.

If the disagreement continued despite discussion, I would avoid arguing or making the issue personal. Instead, I would politely involve a section lead or manager to mediate, ensuring the matter is resolved professionally in a way that supports patient safety and effective teamwork.

Summary:

Disagreements between colleagues are natural, but how they are managed defines professionalism. I believe in handling disagreements through open communication, respect, and evidence-based discussion. Referring to SOPs, guidelines, or involving a senior ensures the right decision is made. The focus should always remain on patient safety, service quality, and maintaining good working relationships, rather than proving who is right. Effective teamwork depends on mutual respect and shared responsibility.

Question 136:

How would you encourage a new member of the team?

Background:

Welcoming and supporting new staff is an important part of maintaining a healthy and productive laboratory environment. New members may feel anxious, unsure, or overwhelmed by new procedures and systems. This question tests your teamwork, leadership, and mentoring skills, as well as how you help others adapt and become confident, competent members of the team.

Points to Consider:

- How to make the new member feel welcome and included.
- Helping them understand lab procedures, culture, and expectations.
- Offering guidance, encouragement, and constructive feedback.
- Encouraging questions and promoting a supportive learning environment.
- Giving practical examples from your experience.

Answer:

When a new member joins the team, I believe the best way to encourage them is through support, communication, and inclusion. Starting a new job can be challenging, especially in a busy laboratory, so I would make an effort to welcome them warmly and help them settle in.

For example, I would introduce myself and other team members, explain how the department is organised, and show them key areas such as sample reception, workbenches, and analyser sections. This helps them feel part of the team from day one.

In Blood Transfusion, I once supported a new Biomedical Scientist who was new to the LIMS system. I encouraged them to shadow me while I processed and issued blood components. I allowed them to ask questions freely and reassured them that it was normal to make mistakes while learning. Over time, I supervised them performing compatibility testing and electronic issue under guidance until they became confident and competent.

In Biochemistry, I helped a new Medical Laboratory Assistant learn the workflow from sample sorting and centrifugation to loading analysers. I encouraged them by acknowledging their progress and giving small responsibilities as their confidence grew. This built trust and motivation.

In Microbiology, I supported a trainee by explaining culture reading and the importance of following SOPs. I shared tips I had learnt from experience and showed them how to document correctly and interpret results under supervision.

In Histopathology, when new staff joined during a busy period, I made sure they were not left behind by pairing them with a mentor or support partner. This allowed them to learn from someone experienced while building confidence with slide tracking, sectioning, and tissue processing procedures.

Overall, I aim to create a friendly environment in which new staff feel comfortable asking questions without fear of judgement.

Encouragement, positive feedback, and patience are essential in building their confidence and supporting their performance.

Summary:

Encouraging a new team member means helping them feel welcomed, valued, and supported. I achieve this by being approachable, patient, and proactive in offering guidance and feedback. By sharing knowledge, promoting teamwork, and recognising their efforts, I help them build confidence and adapt quickly to the laboratory environment. Ultimately, when new staff feel supported, they become productive faster and contribute positively to both team morale and patient care quality.

Question 137:

What is your motivation?

Background:

This question is designed to assess what drives you as a Biomedical Scientist and how your personal and professional motivations align with the role and values of the NHS or laboratory service. The interviewer wants to understand whether your motivation comes from patient care, scientific curiosity, teamwork, professional growth, or a combination of these. Your answer should show passion, purpose, and alignment with the Trust's values such as compassion, respect, improvement, and excellence.

Points to consider:

- Your passion for science, diagnostics, and patient care.
- How your motivation connects to the lab's purpose of supporting patient diagnosis and treatment.
- Examples of situations where your motivation made a difference.
- Long-term motivation, such as career growth, learning new skills, and contributing to service improvement.

Answer:

My motivation comes from knowing that the work I do in the laboratory has a direct and meaningful impact on patient care. Each result I validate contributes to the diagnosis, monitoring, and treatment of patients and that sense of purpose drives me every day.

For example, **in Blood Transfusion**, ensuring that the right blood component is issued promptly and safely to a patient undergoing emergency surgery gives me great satisfaction. **In Haematology**, accurately identifying abnormal blood morphology that helps in diagnosing leukaemia reminds me how crucial our work is to clinicians and patients.

In Biochemistry, processing critical results such as potassium or troponin levels ensures patients receive timely treatment decisions. **In Microbiology,** identifying pathogens correctly allows targeted antibiotic therapy, reducing the risk of complications or hospital-acquired infections. **In Histopathology,** preparing and analysing tissue samples accurately helps in cancer diagnosis and treatment planning.

I am also motivated by opportunities for continuous learning and development. Attending in-house training sessions, completing CPDs, and staying updated with guidelines such as UKAS, MHRA, and ISO15189 requirements help me remain competent and confident in my practice.

In addition, teamwork motivates me. Working with a supportive team where knowledge is shared and every member contributes toward improving patient outcomes creates a positive and inspiring environment. I always feel fulfilled when colleagues collaborate effectively to resolve analytical or quality issues.

Lastly, my motivation comes from improving processes, for example by suggesting workflow changes that reduce turnaround times or improve sample tracking. Seeing these ideas implemented, and knowing they have made a positive difference to patient care, gives me a strong sense of professional achievement.

Summary:

My motivation stems from the desire to provide accurate, timely results that improve patient outcomes, to continue growing professionally, and to contribute positively to the team and the laboratory's quality objectives. The opportunity to make a real difference through science, continuous improvement, and patient-centred service is what inspires me to give my best every day.

Question 138:

How would you keep up to date with your profession?

Background:

Biomedical scientists must remain current with evolving laboratory techniques, best practices, guidelines, and regulatory requirements. Staying up to date ensures safe, accurate, and effective patient care. This question tests your understanding of CPD, professional development, and engagement with scientific advancements.

Points to consider:

- Importance of continuous professional development (CPD)
- Various forms of CPD: academic courses, conferences, workshops, research, competency training
- Following guidelines and regulations (MHRA, BSH, HTA, ISO15189)
- Active participation in professional networks and reading scientific journals
- Practical examples showing engagement with CPD

Answer:

To keep up to date with my profession, I actively engage in a variety of CPD activities. I regularly attend workshops and conferences relevant to my discipline, for example, haematology workshops on new flow cytometry techniques or microbiology webinars on emerging infectious disease diagnostics. I also complete online competency assessments and training modules to reinforce best practices and maintain my registration with the HCPC.

Additionally, I read relevant journals and articles to stay informed about new laboratory techniques, guideline updates, and quality management improvements. For example, I reviewed the latest BSH guidelines for blood transfusion practices and implemented minor workflow adjustments to enhance patient safety. I also participate in in-house training sessions, sharing knowledge with colleagues across departments such as biochemistry, histopathology, and microbiology, to ensure that best practice is applied consistently.

Summary:

I stay up to date with my profession through a combination of formal CPD courses, workshops, online training, scientific reading, and sharing knowledge within the laboratory. This ensures that I remain competent, comply with regulatory standards, and continue to provide accurate and safe laboratory services across all departments.

Question 139:

How do you manage pressure?

Background:

Working in a pathology laboratory can be demanding due to tight turnaround times, high sample volumes, and the critical nature of patient results. Biomedical scientists must be able to manage stress effectively, prioritise workloads, and remain calm to ensure accuracy and patient safety. This question tests your ability to handle pressure, maintain professionalism, and ensure consistent quality under demanding circumstances.

Points to consider:

- Importance of staying calm and composed under pressure
- Time management, prioritisation, and teamwork strategies
- Following SOPs and ensuring accuracy even during high workload periods
- Communicating effectively with colleagues and clinicians
- Giving practical examples in supporting your answer

Answer:

Managing pressure effectively is vital in a laboratory environment, especially when dealing with urgent samples or instrument downtime. I manage pressure by staying calm, prioritising tasks based on clinical urgency, and maintaining clear communication with my team.

For example**, in Haematology**, during peak hours with many urgent samples such as A&E full blood counts and crossmatch requests, I prioritised emergency samples using the laboratory's triage system such as prioritising samples based on urgency, which is not based on the order of sample arrival. For example, I make use of technology or manual review to sort samples based clinical need, while delegating routine work to other team members. By keeping communication open and following SOPs, we ensured timely and accurate reporting without compromising quality.

In Biochemistry, when the analyser once broke down during a busy morning shift, I immediately informed the senior scientist, performed manual testing for critical electrolytes, and liaised with the engineer for urgent maintenance. At the same time, I communicated with the wards about expected delays and alternative processing options.

Outside of direct bench work, I manage pressure by maintaining good organisation. This includes preparing reagents in advance, keeping a clean workspace, and using checklists to ensure that nothing is overlooked.

Summary:

I manage pressure by staying calm, prioritising tasks, following SOPs, and maintaining clear communication with colleagues and clinicians. Whether working alone or as part of a team, I focus on patient safety and quality, ensuring deadlines are met without compromising accuracy. This balanced approach allows me to remain effective and dependable, even in high-pressure laboratory environments.

Question 140:

What would you do to improve patient care?

Background:

Patient care is at the centre of biomedical science practice. Every test performed in the laboratory contributes to diagnosis, treatment, and monitoring of patients. Improving patient care involves maintaining high analytical standards, ensuring timely results, reducing pre-analytical and post-analytical errors, effective communication with clinical teams, and continuous quality improvement. This question tests your understanding of how laboratory practices directly affect patient outcomes and what actions you can take to enhance that impact.

Points to consider:

- The link between laboratory work and patient outcomes
- Accuracy, reliability, and timeliness of results
- Quality assurance, training, and communication
- Error prevention and process improvement
- Collaboration with clinical teams

Answer:

Improving patient care begins with ensuring accuracy, reliability, and timeliness of laboratory results. I focus on following standard operating procedures, performing daily quality control checks, and validating results carefully before release.

For example, **in Haematology**, I ensure urgent samples such as suspected leukaemia are processed and reviewed promptly so clinicians can initiate treatment quickly. **In Biochemistry,** I check for sample integrity issues such as haemolysis, lipaemia, or insufficient volume, and request repeats when necessary to ensure that the results provided are clinically valid.

In Microbiology, I contribute to patient care by ensuring that cultures are read promptly, sensitivity results are verified, and significant findings are communicated quickly to the infection control or clinical teams. Similarly, **in Histopathology**, timely embedding, sectioning, and staining of urgent biopsies helps consultant's report cases faster, leading to early treatment decisions.

Beyond the bench, I also promote patient care by maintaining good communication with colleagues and clinicians, participating in audit and quality improvement projects, and engaging in continuous professional development to stay updated with best practices.

Summary:

I improve patient care by ensuring the accuracy and timeliness of results, following SOPs, maintaining effective communication, and supporting quality improvement initiatives. Whether through daily analytical work or broader service enhancement, my goal is to contribute to safe, efficient, and high-quality laboratory services that directly support patient diagnosis and treatment.

Question 141:

You received 3 emergency/equally critical requests while at work alone on a night duty. How would you manage it?

Background:

Biomedical scientists often face high-pressure situations, especially during out-of-hours (OOH) shifts, where multiple urgent requests arrive simultaneously. Timely decision-making, prioritisation based on patient safety, adherence to SOPs, and clear communication with clinical teams are critical to prevent harm. This question tests your ability to manage competing emergencies efficiently while maintaining accuracy.

Points to consider:

- Assess urgency and life-threatening potential of each request
- Prioritise tasks that directly impact immediate patient survival
- Effective time and workflow management
- Communication with clinical teams to manage expectations
- Adherence to SOPs and quality standards
- Practical examples from specific departments

Answer:

If I receive three emergency requests at the same time on a night shift, I will first quickly assess which request is most life-threatening.

Example in Haematology/Blood Transfusion:

Scenario: I receive urgent blood for a massive haemorrhage in theatre, an urgent crossmatch for a critically ill patient in A&E, and a request to process a STAT sample for a severely anaemic patient in the ward.

Step 1 - Prioritisation: I immediately identify the massive haemorrhage patient as the highest risk, as any delay could be fatal. I focus on issuing compatible blood units first.

Step 2 - Delegate or stagger: While I am issuing the blood, I alert the ward team that the crossmatch and STAT sample will be processed as soon as possible. If there is any task that can be safely prepared in parallel (like setting up a centrifuge or checking patient ID), I do that while issuing blood.

Step 3 - Sequential handling: Once the most critical blood transfusion is completed and the units delivered, I immediately process the crossmatch for the second patient, ensuring all checks are done accurately. Finally, I address the STAT anaemia sample.

Example in Biochemistry:

Scenario: Three critical chemistry samples arrive: suspected hyperkalaemia in ICU, suspected sepsis patient requiring lactate measurement, and acute liver failure sample.

Step 1 - Life-threatening first: I start with hyperkalaemia because immediate intervention can prevent cardiac arrest.

Step 2 - Parallel preparation: I set up the analyser for the sepsis sample and ensure all reagents are ready while waiting for hyperkalaemia result.

Step 3 - Sequential handling: Once the potassium result is reported, I quickly process lactate, then the liver function tests, maintaining clear documentation throughout.

Example in Microbiology:

Scenario: Blood cultures from a septic patient, a urine sample from a patient with suspected urosepsis, and a CSF from suspected meningitis arrive simultaneously.

Step 1 - Prioritise highest immediate risk: I process the CSF first as delay could have serious consequences, inoculate culture media and send alert to the clinical team.

Step 2 - Process the other blood cultures next, followed by the urine sample, keeping clinicians updated on expected turnaround times.

Summary:

In high-pressure situations where multiple emergencies occur at once, I prioritise based on immediate patient risk. Life-threatening requests are always handled first. I use a combination of rapid assessment, sequential task management, and efficient use of any preparatory or parallel steps to ensure all requests are completed accurately. Communication with the clinical teams is maintained

throughout to manage expectations and safeguard patient safety. This approach ensures that urgent results are delivered in a timely manner without compromising quality or accuracy, whether in haematology, blood transfusion, biochemistry, microbiology, or histopathology.

Question 142:

Tell us about your professional experience from beginning till now.

Background:

This question allows you to demonstrate your career journey, highlighting your progression, skills, and experiences. It tests your ability to articulate your professional development, show alignment with the Biomedical Scientist role, and indicate how your previous experience will benefit the Trust.

Points to consider:

- Start from academic qualifications and early experience
- Include previous roles in laboratory or related healthcare positions
- Highlight progression, responsibilities, and skills gained
- Mention any specialised experience across different pathology departments
- Use practical examples to show competency

Answer:

I began my professional journey with a degree in Biomedical Science, where I gained foundational knowledge in haematology, biochemistry, microbiology, and immunology. During my academic training, I completed placements that introduced me to routine laboratory practices, quality control, and SOP adherence.

After graduation, I started as a Band 5 Biomedical Scientist in a busy NHS laboratory. Initially, I focused on performing routine tests under supervision, such as full blood counts in haematology and clinical chemistry panels in biochemistry. I developed competence in sample processing, analyser operation, and result validation.

Over time, I progressed to handling more complex tasks independently. In blood transfusion, I performed crossmatches and issued compatible units, ensuring patient safety through strict adherence to LIMS and SOPs. In microbiology, I processed blood cultures and supported the identification of pathogenic organisms, using both automated systems and manual techniques while maintaining required turnaround times. In histopathology, I assisted with tissue processing and staining, ensuring accurate sample tracking and thorough documentation.

Alongside technical skills, I have been actively involved in quality management. I participate in internal and external quality control schemes, contribute to audit activities, and help train junior staff. I have also supported laboratory service improvements, such as streamlining sample workflows and introducing minor procedural adjustments that improved turnaround times.

I continue to undertake CPD, including academic courses, training workshops, and attending relevant conferences. This has helped me stay up to date with regulatory requirements, ISO15189 standards, and evolving laboratory technologies.

Summary:

My professional experience spans from academic training to independent work across multiple pathology disciplines, including haematology, blood transfusion, biochemistry, microbiology, and histopathology. I have developed technical competence, problem-solving skills, and leadership abilities, while contributing to quality management and service improvement. This experience has equipped me to work efficiently, safely, and collaboratively, making me well-prepared for the Biomedical Scientist role in your Trust.

Question 143:

Who do you think our customers are?

Background:

Laboratory services rely on both internal and external customers to ensure effective patient care. Understanding who your customers are shows awareness of your role within the wider healthcare system and the importance of meeting their needs. This question tests your understanding of stakeholders and how your work contributes to patient care.

Points to consider:

- Identify internal and external customers
- Highlight how laboratory services support their work
- Use practical examples to show understanding of customer impact

Answer:

In a pathology laboratory, our customers are both internal and external. Internally, this includes clinicians, nurses, and other healthcare professionals who rely on accurate and timely test results to make clinical decisions. For example, **in haematology**, accurate full blood counts or coagulation results are essential for clinicians managing acutely unwell patients. **In microbiology**, rapid identification of pathogens allows infection teams to prescribe the correct antibiotics.

Externally, patients are also key customers because laboratory results directly affect their diagnosis, treatment, and overall care. For instance, **in blood transfusion**, ensuring the correct blood group match and issuing compatible units safely directly impacts patient outcomes during surgery or emergency transfusions.

Other customers can include researchers, public health bodies, and regulatory agencies who rely on laboratory data to support studies, audits, and compliance. For example, providing accurate data for an external quality assessment or reporting surveillance data to public health authorities ensures wider patient safety.

Summary:

I understand that a laboratory's customers include internal stakeholders like clinicians, nurses, and other healthcare professionals, as well as external stakeholders such as patients, researchers, and regulatory bodies. Meeting their needs through accurate, timely, and reliable results is central to laboratory service, patient safety, and overall healthcare delivery.

Question 144:

Where are you at in your career?

Background:

This question assesses your self-awareness, reflection on career progress, and your future aspirations. It helps interviewers understand your motivation, career trajectory, and readiness for the role.

Points to consider:

- Highlight your current level of experience and skills
- Reflect on your achievements and growth
- Show ambition and alignment with the new role
- Give examples of progression or learning opportunities

Answer:

At this stage in my career, I am an experienced Biomedical Scientist with a strong foundation across multiple pathology disciplines, including haematology, biochemistry, microbiology, and blood transfusion. I have gained substantial hands-on experience with routine and complex analyses, equipment operation, quality management systems, and compliance with ISO15189 standards.

For example, **in biochemistry,** I have managed high-volume testing while ensuring accuracy and turnaround times. **In blood transfusion**, I have participated in both routine crossmatches and emergency major haemorrhage protocols, ensuring patient safety and timely blood issuance. I have also mentored junior staff, supported CPD activities, and contributed to laboratory audits and quality improvements.

Currently, I am focused on consolidating my leadership and specialist skills, taking on responsibilities that allow me to contribute to service improvements, process optimisation, and team development. I am also actively maintaining my CPD portfolio to stay updated with advancements in laboratory science.

Summary:

I see myself as an experienced Biomedical Scientist ready to take on more responsibility, contribute to team development, and enhance laboratory services. My career progression reflects both technical competence and leadership growth, and I am eager to apply my skills to make a meaningful impact in this role.

Question 145:

What do you think this role involves, and why did you apply for it

Background:

This question assesses your understanding of the role, its responsibilities, and your motivation for applying. Interviewers want to see that you know what the job entails and that your skills, experience, and interests align with the position.

Points to consider:

- Demonstrate understanding of the role's duties
- Link your experience and skills to the role
- Show enthusiasm and motivation for applying
- Highlight how the role fits your career goals

Answer:

I understand that this Biomedical Scientist role involves providing high-quality diagnostic laboratory services across various disciplines, such as haematology, biochemistry, microbiology, and blood transfusion. The role includes processing and analysing patient samples, ensuring results are accurate and delivered within the required turnaround times, maintaining compliance with ISO15189 and other regulatory standards, participating in quality management systems, and supporting continuous improvement initiatives. It also involves mentoring junior staff, contributing to audits, and maintaining competence through CPD.

I applied for this role because it aligns perfectly with my skills, experience, and career ambitions. I am motivated by the opportunity to contribute to patient care by delivering accurate and timely results, supporting laboratory quality improvement, and developing professionally within a multidisciplinary team environment. For example, in my previous role, I successfully managed complex blood transfusion cases and high-volume biochemistry workloads, which has prepared me to take on the responsibilities this role requires.

Summary:

This role involves delivering accurate and timely laboratory services, maintaining high standards of quality, and contributing to team and service development. I applied because it matches my experience and career goals, and I am motivated to contribute to patient care, laboratory quality, and professional growth

Question 146:

What do you think you can bring to the lab here

Background:

This question assesses your ability to reflect on your strengths, experience, and personal attributes that will add value to the laboratory and the wider Trust. It also evaluates your understanding of how your contribution aligns with the organisation's goals, values, and commitment to patient centred service delivery.

Points to consider:

- Identify specific skills, knowledge, and attributes you offer
- Link your contribution to service improvement and patient care
- Mention teamwork, quality, innovation, and professionalism
- Use practical examples to support your answer.

Answer:

I believe I can bring a combination of technical expertise, commitment to quality, and a strong sense of teamwork to the laboratory. My experience across haematology, biochemistry, blood transfusion, microbiology, and histopathology has equipped me with a broad understanding of laboratory processes and interdepartmental collaboration.

For example, **in haematology**, I have developed strong analytical and troubleshooting skills, particularly when working under pressure during analyser downtime or when validating complex results. **In blood transfusion**, I have demonstrated meticulous attention to detail when crossmatching and issuing blood components during major haemorrhage protocols by ensuring accuracy and patient safety. **In biochemistry**, I have contributed to process improvement by reviewing sample rejection trends and suggesting ways to reduce pre-analytical errors through clearer communication with clinical areas.

Beyond technical skills, I bring a positive attitude and a willingness to support colleagues. I believe in open communication, sharing knowledge, and maintaining a culture of continuous improvement. My focus on compliance with ISO15189 standards and QMS processes ensures that all work meets regulatory and professional expectations.

Summary:

I bring technical competence, quality-focused work ethics, and a collaborative mindset to the laboratory. My broad experience across pathology disciplines allows me to adapt quickly, maintain accuracy under pressure, and contribute positively to patient-centred service delivery. I am dedicated to supporting both the team's performance and the Trust's commitment to safe, efficient, and high-quality laboratory services.

Question 147:

What support will you need from us if you are successful in this role

Background:

This question is testing your self-awareness, understanding of your professional development needs, and ability to identify what support will help you succeed in the new role. It also helps the panel assess how well you can integrate into the team and what kind of management or mentoring structure will best support your growth.

Points to consider:

- Acknowledge the importance of a good induction and mentorship
- Identify realistic support needs (training, feedback, resources, etc.)
- Show willingness to learn and integrate into the team
- Relate support to professional development and patient care
- Use practical examples from previous experiences

Answer:

If I am successful in this role, the support I would need primarily relates to a structured induction, clear guidance, and mentorship to ensure I integrate smoothly into the team and fully understand the Trust's systems and expectations.

For example, I would appreciate an initial orientation period to familiarise myself with the laboratory layout, equipment, LIMS system, and any local procedures that may differ from my previous experience. Every Trust can have slight variations in processes or analysers even for similar tests. So, understanding these local protocols will help me work efficiently and maintain quality from the start.

I would also value ongoing feedback and mentorship from senior colleagues, especially during the first few months. For example, in my previous role in haematology, I benefited greatly from weekly check-ins with a senior biomedical scientist who reviewed my validation approach and provided practical advice on complex cases. That kind of structured feedback helped me grow in confidence and improve my accuracy.

Additionally, I would appreciate opportunities for continued professional development (CPD) through in-house training sessions, external courses, or multidisciplinary meetings. For example, attending Trust-wide quality or audit meetings would help me understand the broader perspective of laboratory service delivery and patient care.

Summary:

The key support I would need includes a structured induction, access to mentorship, regular feedback, and opportunities for continuous professional development. These will help me adapt quickly, uphold laboratory standards, and contribute effectively to patient safety and service quality. In return, I am committed to being proactive, open to learning, and adding value to the laboratory team from day one.

Question 148:

What's your understanding of diversity, and tell me when you have demonstrated this

Background:

This question is testing your awareness of equality, diversity, and inclusion (EDI) and how you apply these principles in the workplace. In the NHS, diversity is not only about respecting differences in race, gender, age, religion, disability, or sexual orientation but also about recognising and valuing everyone's unique contribution to patient care and teamwork.

You are expected to show that you:

- Understand the importance of diversity in healthcare
- Treat colleagues and patients with fairness and respect
- Demonstrate inclusive behaviour in real-life situations
- Contribute to creating a supportive and respectful workplace culture

Answer:

Diversity, to me, means recognising, respecting, and valuing people's differences, whether in background, culture, beliefs, skills, or perspectives, and ensuring that everyone feels included and treated fairly. In a laboratory or healthcare setting, diversity also extends to how we interact with patients and colleagues to deliver safe, equitable, and respectful care.

I have demonstrated my understanding of diversity in my daily practice by working collaboratively with colleagues from different cultural, religious, and professional backgrounds. For example, while working **in the haematology and blood transfusion laboratory**, we had a multidisciplinary team of scientists, assistants, and doctors from different parts of the world. I always made an effort to communicate respectfully, listen to different viewpoints, and adapt my approach when explaining a complex issue especially when language barriers or different communication styles were involved.

Another example was during a training session with a new member of staff whose first language was not English. I noticed that they were hesitant to ask questions, so I took the time to demonstrate procedures more slowly and encouraged them to shadow me until they felt confident. This approach helped the staff member settle in quickly and feel valued as part of the team, which in turn improved teamwork and accuracy on shift.

I also respect diversity in religious and cultural practices. For instance, I have offered to adjust work schedules during Ramadan or Christmas to accommodate colleagues observing religious commitments. Small gestures like this promote understanding and strengthen team cohesion.

Summary:

My understanding of diversity is about treating everyone with respect, fairness, and understanding, while appreciating the value that different backgrounds bring to the workplace. I demonstrate this by fostering open communication, being supportive of others' needs, and encouraging an inclusive, collaborative environment where everyone feels valued and able to contribute fully to patient care.

Question 149:

Tell us a time When you had to work under pressure, how did you cope and what you learnt.

Background:

In laboratory settings, pressure can arise from emergency samples, equipment failure, high workloads, or staff shortages. This question assesses your ability to stay calm, prioritise tasks, and maintain quality and accuracy under demanding situations. Interviewers also want to see reflection what you learnt and how it improved your practice.

You are expected to show that you:

- Can manage stress effectively without compromising patient safety.
- Use prioritisation, communication, and teamwork under pressure.
- Reflect on the experience and identify lessons learned.
- Understand the importance of SOPs, time management, and escalation when needed.

Answer:

Working under pressure is an essential part of being a Biomedical Scientist, as timely and accurate results are often critical to patient care.

For example, during an out-of-hours shift in Blood Transfusion, we received a major haemorrhage call from the emergency department while I was already processing urgent crossmatches for obstetric and surgical patients. I remained calm and prioritised according to clinical urgency. The trauma case was the most life-threatening, so I initiated the Massive Haemorrhage Protocol (MHP), selected appropriate emergency O-negative blood units, and ensured that the sample for crossmatching was fast-tracked. I kept the communication line open with clinicians and colleagues, and while I handled the crossmatching, another colleague helped with packaging and issuing the blood. Once the situation was stabilised, I returned to complete the other pending tasks.

In Haematology, I have also faced pressure when multiple analysers failed simultaneously during peak hours. I immediately informed the duty manager, began manual differential and film reviews for the most critical requests (such as A&E and ITU samples), and ensured communication with wards about expected delays. This ensured urgent results were still provided promptly and safely.

Similarly, **in Microbiology**, during a COVID-19 surge, sample numbers increased significantly. I managed pressure by batching samples efficiently, using downtime protocols, and communicating with clinicians on prioritisation, particularly for intensive care and theatre patients.

Summary:

Working under pressure requires composure, clear prioritisation, and teamwork. I have learned that maintaining calmness and clear communication is key. Using established protocols, seeking support when necessary, and focusing on patient safety help ensure quality even under demanding conditions. These experiences have strengthened my ability to stay organised, adaptable, and dependable essential qualities for any Biomedical Scientist.

Question 150:

Tell us about a mistake you made and what you have learnt from it

Background:

Mistakes can happen in any professional setting, including laboratory practice. What matters most is how one responds by identifying the cause, taking corrective actions, reporting the incident appropriately, and applying lessons learned to prevent recurrence. This question tests honesty, accountability, and professional maturity.

You are expected to show that you:

- Take responsibility for your actions and follow the correct reporting procedure.
- Understand the importance of learning from errors and preventing future recurrence.
- Maintain patient safety and professional standards at all times.
- Communicate openly and demonstrate reflection.

Answer:

In the laboratory, accuracy and attention to detail are crucial. Early in my career, I once booked a sample in Haematology under the wrong patient's name due to similar patient identifiers. Fortunately, I identified the error during result validation before the report was released. I immediately followed the laboratory's incident reporting procedure, informed my senior colleague, corrected the record, and documented the event through the non-conformance system.

This experience reminded me of the importance of carefully checking three patient identifiers name, date of birth, and hospital or NHS number before booking in or validating results. Since then, I have made it a strict habit to double-check every sample entry and encourage colleagues to do the same.

In another instance, in Blood Transfusion, I once noticed I had nearly selected the wrong blood unit during issue because two similar patient surnames appeared close together on LIMS. I stopped, rechecked the details, and realised the potential mistake before it occurred. This reinforced to me how easy it is to make errors under time pressure and why slowing down to check is essential even in emergencies.

Summary:

I have learned that mistakes are opportunities to improve. Being honest, taking responsibility, and following proper reporting procedures protect both patients and staff. Each time an error happens or nearly happens. I reflect on what caused it and apply preventive measures. This experience has helped me become more vigilant, confident, and committed to maintaining a culture of safety and quality in the laboratory.

Question 151:

What factors will you consider when introducing a new test or machine?

Background:

Introducing a new test or analyser in a pathology laboratory requires careful planning to ensure accuracy, reliability, cost-effectiveness, and patient safety. This process is part of the laboratory's Quality Management System (QMS) and must comply with UKAS, HTA and MHRA requirements. The question tests your understanding of quality assurance, validation, training, and the practical steps needed for implementation.

You are expected to show that you:

- Understand validation, verification, and correlation processes.
- Recognise the importance of training, documentation, and SOP updates.
- Consider patient impact, workflow efficiency, and cost.
- Understand regulatory and quality compliance requirements.

Answer:

When introducing a new test or analyser, I would first consider clinical need and justification for the new test or analyser. For example, understanding why the new equipment or test should be introduced and how it improves patient care.

Next, I would consider method verification or validation, ensuring the new system produces accurate, reliable, and reproducible results compared with the current method or a reference standard. For example, in Haematology, if introducing a new full blood count analyser, I would perform parallel testing with existing analysers to confirm result comparability.

Training and competency are equally important. I would ensure that all the required staff receive adequate training on the new system and demonstrate competency before independent use. For example, in Blood Transfusion, when introducing a new blood tracking system, every user must be trained on how to issue and return blood safely within the new software environment.

Quality control (IQC/EQA) must be established before live use to ensure ongoing performance monitoring. Similarly, SOPs and risk assessments must be updated or newly written to reflect the new process.

I would also consider cost and maintenance requirements, ensuring value for money, easy access to consumables, and technical support availability.

Lastly, communication and collaboration are crucial, involving clinicians, the laboratory manager, and the quality team throughout to ensure a smooth transition. For example, in biochemistry, introducing a new troponin assay would require coordination with the A&E department to update clinical decision limits and reporting thresholds.

Summary:

When introducing a new test or analyser, I consider clinical relevance, validation, training, documentation, and quality assurance as top priorities. Involving the right stakeholders, following standard verification processes, and ensuring staff competence help maintain accuracy, safety, and efficiency. Ultimately, any new system must support reliable patient results and continuous improvement in laboratory service delivery.

Question 152:

What does team work mean to you and give example where you have been a good team member?

Background:

Teamwork is essential in the laboratory environment because it ensures smooth workflow, accuracy, and timely delivery of results that directly impact patient care. This question tests your understanding of what teamwork means in practice and how your contribution supports the success of the team.

You are expected to show that you:

- Understand the importance of teamwork in a clinical laboratory.
- Can work collaboratively with colleagues at all levels.
- Communicate effectively and support others when under pressure.
- Can provide a real-life example that demonstrates your teamwork skills.

Answer:

To me, teamwork means working collaboratively with others to achieve a common goal, supporting one another to ensure quality, accuracy, and efficiency in laboratory operations. It involves communication, respect, reliability, and flexibility, knowing when to lead and when to support.

For example, **in Blood Transfusion,** during a busy night shift, we received several urgent requests for blood units from different wards, including A&E and maternity. While one colleague was preparing the crossmatch, I checked the patient details on LIMS, confirmed compatibility, and ensured the issue documentation was completed. Another colleague helped with packaging and transport coordination. By sharing responsibilities and communicating clearly, we were able to meet the urgent requests safely and on time.

Similarly**, in Haematology,** when the main analyser broke down, the entire team came together to manage samples manually. I assisted in performing manual differential counts while others re-ran urgent samples on a backup analyser. We prioritised emergency samples and informed the wards of expected turnaround times. This experience showed how teamwork can turn a stressful situation into an organised and safe response.

In Microbiology, teamwork was equally vital. During a high number of culture-positive cases, I assisted colleagues in reading plates and verifying results, ensuring no backlog. We discussed findings collectively before authorising reports to ensure consistency and accuracy.

In Histopathology, teamwork is just as important. During a time when the tissue processor malfunctioned, we worked together to manage the backlog. For example, I assisted in embedding and labelling cassettes, while others prepared slides and ensured urgent biopsies were prioritised. This collaboration prevented significant delays in patient diagnosis.

Summary:

Teamwork, to me, means shared responsibility and mutual support to achieve reliable, timely, and safe results. I believe in communicating openly, offering help when others are under pressure, and contributing positively to the workflow. Through experiences in departments like Blood Transfusion, Haematology, and Microbiology, I have learned that effective teamwork not only reduces stress but also enhances patient safety and laboratory efficiency.

Question 153:

What is quality control and quality assurance?

Background:

Quality Control (QC) and Quality Assurance (QA) are two essential components of the laboratory Quality Management System (QMS) that ensure accuracy, reliability, and consistency of test results. While both aim to maintain quality, they work at different levels. QC checks the performance of the test process, and QA ensures the overall system supports consistent quality outcomes.

You are expected to show that you:

- Understand the difference between QC and QA.

- Can link both concepts to ISO 15189 requirements.
- Appreciate their roles in maintaining accurate, reliable laboratory results.
- Use practical examples that support your answer.

Answer:

Quality Control (QC) is a day-to-day operational process that ensures the test system is performing within acceptable limits. It involves running control materials of known values alongside patient samples to monitor the analyser's performance, reagent integrity, and staff technique.

For example, **in Haematology,** internal QC samples are run at the start of each shift to verify that the full blood count analyser produces accurate results. If the QC result is out of range, the test run is stopped, the problem is investigated (such as recalibration or reagent replacement), and patient results are not released until the issue is resolved.

In Blood Transfusion, QC ensures that blood grouping reagents and crossmatching methods are performing correctly. For example, running positive and negative control samples each day to confirm reagent reliability.

In Biochemistry, QC checks are performed for each analyte (e.g., sodium, potassium, glucose) using low, normal, and high control levels to ensure linearity and precision.

In Microbiology, QC may include checking the performance of culture media or antibiotic discs using known control organisms to confirm expected growth or inhibition patterns.

Quality Assurance (QA), on the other hand, is a broader, system-wide process that ensures the entire laboratory system consistently produces accurate and reliable results. It covers pre-analytical, analytical, and post-analytical stages like from sample collection, processing, and analysis to result reporting.

QA includes:

- Document control and SOP management (ensuring everyone follows standardised procedures).
- Participation in External Quality Assessment (EQA) schemes to compare laboratory performance with other labs.
- Internal audits to check compliance with standards such as ISO 15189.
- Training and competency assessments for all staff.

For example, **in Histopathology,** QA includes double-reporting of critical diagnoses (e.g., malignancy) and slide peer reviews to maintain diagnostic accuracy. **In Microbiology,** it includes participation in national EQA schemes for antimicrobial susceptibility testing to ensure results are consistent with national standards.

Summary:

In simple terms, Quality Control ensures accuracy on the bench, while Quality Assurance ensures consistency across the entire laboratory system. QC focuses on identifying and correcting problems in real time, while QA ensures that the processes, training, documentation, and audits are in place to prevent such issues. Both QC and QA work together under the Quality Management System (QMS) to ensure patient results are accurate, reliable, and meet ISO 15189 standards and ultimately safeguarding patient care and laboratory integrity.

Question 154:

Aside bench work, what else do you do in your current position?

Background:

While bench work forms the core of a Biomedical Scientist's role, laboratories rely on additional non-analytical responsibilities to maintain quality, safety, and efficiency. This question tests your understanding of the wider laboratory responsibilities beyond sample testing such as quality management, audits, training, equipment maintenance, and continuous improvement activities, which are vital under ISO 15189 and UKAS accreditation.

You are expected to show that you:

- Understand that Biomedical Science involves more than analytical bench work.
- Can demonstrate involvement in quality, training, health and safety, and process improvement.
- Use practical examples to support your answer.
- Reflect how your wider contribution aligns with Trust or departmental goals.

Answer:

Aside from bench work, I am actively involved in several non-analytical responsibilities that support the overall quality and efficiency of the laboratory.

Firstly, I take part in quality management activities such as reviewing and updating SOPs, logging non-conformances, and participating in internal audits to maintain compliance with ISO 15189 and UKAS standards. For example, in my department, I helped review the sample rejection policy after noticing recurring pre-analytical errors, which led to improved communication with wards and reduced sample rejections.

I am also involved in training and competency assessment. For example, I support Band 5 Biomedical Scientists and trainee staff by demonstrating bench techniques, observing their performance, and providing feedback in line with competency assessment frameworks.

Another important aspect of my role is equipment and analyser management, which includes performing and documenting daily, weekly, and monthly maintenance tasks, ensuring calibration logs are kept up to date, and reporting faults to the senior BMS or engineer. For example, in biochemistry, I have supported the documentation of analyser downtime investigations to help maintain service continuity and contribute to root cause analysis.

In Blood Transfusion, I participate in EQA reviews, checking for performance trends and ensuring that corrective actions are implemented and documented appropriately.

I am also part of the Health and Safety team, contributing to risk assessments and ensuring COSHH forms are up to date, especially when new reagents or chemicals are introduced.

Additionally, I contribute to CPD activities by attending webinars, training sessions, and trust-wide meetings and I record all my CPD on the IBMS portal to maintain my HCPC registration.

Finally, I am involved in continuous improvement projects. For example, I recently contributed to improving sample turnaround times by suggesting workflow changes during peak periods, which helped redistribute workload more effectively among team members.

Summary:

In addition to bench duties, I actively support quality management, training, equipment maintenance, safety, and service improvement initiatives. These tasks ensure the laboratory operates smoothly, complies with ISO 15189 standards, and delivers accurate, timely, and reliable results. I believe that combining technical and non-technical responsibilities is key to maintaining excellence and continuous improvement in the laboratory.

Question 155:

What is a near miss and what do you do about it?

Background:

A near miss is an event that could have led to an adverse outcome, such as patient harm, equipment failure, or safety breach, but was identified and corrected before any damage occurred. In the pathology laboratory, near misses are important indicators of potential risks and are vital for continuous improvement under ISO 15189, UKAS, and HCPC standards. This question tests your understanding of identifying, reporting, and learning from near misses to maintain patient safety and laboratory quality.

You are expected to show that you:

- Understand what constitutes a near miss in the laboratory setting.
- Recognise the importance of reporting and documenting near misses.
- Demonstrate how you would investigate and learn from such incidents.
- Give practical examples that supports your answer.

Answer:

A near miss is an incident that could have caused an error or patient harm but was detected and corrected before affecting the final result or outcome. It represents a valuable opportunity to identify weaknesses in our systems and prevent future errors.

When a near miss occurs, my first step is to make the situation safe and correct any immediate issue if possible. Then I document and report the incident through the laboratory's Quality Management System (such as Q-Pulse or Datix) as a non-conformance or near-miss report. This allows the senior BMS or quality officer to investigate, determine the root cause, and implement corrective and preventive actions (CAPA).

For example, **in Haematology**, a sample was nearly reported under the wrong patient ID because two tubes had similar identifiers. I spotted the discrepancy during LIMS verification and stopped the process immediately. I logged the event on Q-Pulse as a near miss, and we later reviewed the sample labelling policy with the phlebotomy team to prevent a recurrence.

In Blood Transfusion, I once noticed a discrepancy between the patient's date of birth on the blood bag and the request form during issue. I stopped the issue process, double-checked on LIMS, and confirmed it was a transcription error. This was reported as a near miss, investigated, and discussed in the departmental meeting. It led to a reminder to always perform the three-point check (patient name, date of birth, hospital number) before issuing any blood product.

In Biochemistry, a reagent bottle was nearly used beyond its expiry date. I noticed the date during a reagent change, quarantined the bottle, and informed the senior scientist. The near miss was reported, and expiry date verification became part of the pre-use checklist to strengthen quality control.

In Microbiology, near misses might involve plating samples on incorrect media or delayed incubation. Identifying and correcting these before result release prevents inaccurate organism identification or missed growth.

Summary:

A near miss is an event that could have caused an error or harm but was caught in time. I treat near misses as opportunities to learn, review, and strengthen laboratory processes. By reporting them promptly, investigating root causes, and implementing corrective actions, we uphold ISO 15189 standards, maintain UKAS compliance, and most importantly, protect patient safety.

Question 156:

What is the difference between an accredited lab and a non-accredited lab?

Background:

In the UK, medical laboratories are assessed against ISO 15189:2022 standards by the United Kingdom Accreditation Service (UKAS). Accreditation confirms that a lab operates with robust quality management, technical competence, and consistent standards in testing. Understanding the difference between accredited and non-accredited laboratories is essential for ensuring patient safety, traceability, and compliance with regulatory and professional expectations.

You are expected to show that you:

- Understand what laboratory accreditation means and why it matters.
- Can explain the practical implications of accreditation on patient safety, reliability, and trust.
- Can differentiate between accredited and non-accredited labs using real-world examples.

Answer:

An accredited laboratory is one that has been formally assessed and approved by UKAS to meet the requirements of ISO 15189:2022 for medical laboratories. Accreditation demonstrates that the laboratory has the necessary technical competence, quality management system, and consistent procedures to produce reliable, traceable, and valid results.

In contrast, a non-accredited laboratory may still perform diagnostic testing, but its processes and results have not been independently verified against international standards. This means there is no formal assurance that the lab consistently meets defined levels of quality, accuracy, and safety.

In an accredited lab, strict quality control and assurance measures are in place such as:

- Use of validated methods and equipment.
- Participation in Internal Quality Control (IQC) and External Quality Assurance (EQA) schemes.
- Documented Standard Operating Procedures (SOPs) and adherence to traceability and audit trails.
- Continuous review through internal audits, management review meetings, and corrective/preventive actions (CAPA).

These ensure that patient results are consistent, reproducible, and trustworthy across time and locations.

For example, in a UKAS-accredited **Haematology or Biochemistry laboratory**, each analyser and test method is validated and regularly reviewed. If a control fails, results are withheld until investigation is completed ensuring patient safety. Similarly, **in Microbiology and Histopathology,** all stains, cultures, and procedures are monitored through quality checks, and deviations are documented and investigated.

In a non-accredited laboratory, some of these processes may be informal or applied inconsistently. For example, IQC and EQA may not be performed regularly, and there may be no robust documentation system to track instrument performance or corrective actions. This increases the risk of unreliable results, non-traceable practices, and reduced confidence in patient care decisions.

Summary:

The main difference is that an accredited laboratory operates under a formally recognised quality and competence framework, while a non-accredited laboratory lacks that independent verification. Accreditation ensures confidence, traceability, and consistency in testing, supporting patient

safety and regulatory compliance. Working in an accredited lab gives assurance that all processes meet internationally accepted standards, helping maintain high-quality diagnostic outcomes.

Question 157:

What will you do when you see your colleague doing the wrong thing in the lab?

Background:

Working in a pathology laboratory demands strict adherence to Standard Operating Procedures (SOPs), Health and Safety, and Quality Management System (QMS) policies. Any deviation whether intentional or accidental can affect patient results, safety, and the laboratory's accreditation. This question tests your professional integrity, communication skills, and commitment to patient safety by assessing how you would handle an incident where a colleague acts incorrectly.

You are expected to show that you:

- Understand the importance of raising concerns professionally and safely.
- Can act in a way that promotes a just culture - focusing on learning, not blame.
- Know how to use the appropriate reporting channels (senior staff, Quality Officer, or Datix).
- Appreciate the balance between team relationships and professional accountability.

Answer:

If I observed a colleague doing something wrong in the laboratory, my first response would be to act professionally, calmly, and discreetly, ensuring patient safety remains the top priority.

If the issue is minor or procedural, such as forgetting to label a sample correctly or bypassing an SOP step unintentionally, I would politely intervene and offer to assist or remind them of the correct process. For example, **in Haematology**, if I notice a colleague attempting to release results before QC validation, I will stop the process and remind them to check the control first.

However, if the mistake is serious or could affect patient safety such as issuing the wrong blood unit **in Transfusion**, mislabelling a specimen **in Histopathology**, or overriding an analyser flag **in Biochemistry**, I would immediately stop the process and escalate the matter to the senior biomedical scientist or shift lead. I would also document the incident through the appropriate incident reporting system (e.g. Datix) to ensure it is investigated and used as a learning opportunity.

In Microbiology, for example, if I saw a colleague disposing of cultures incorrectly, I would intervene to prevent contamination or infection risk, then raise the issue with the department safety officer for follow-up.

My approach would always be non-confrontational by focusing on the procedure, not the person. I would remember that everyone can make mistakes and that a supportive environment encourages openness and improvement rather than blame.

Summary:

When a colleague does something wrong in the lab, I would act professionally and promptly to prevent patient harm, correct the mistake, and report it appropriately. I would address the issue respectfully, follow escalation procedures, and use the event as an opportunity for shared learning. This approach supports a just culture, reinforces team accountability, and upholds the integrity of laboratory practice.

Question 158:

How do you reflect our trust values?

Background:

Every NHS Trust has a set of core values that guide behaviour, teamwork, and patient care. While the specific wording may differ between Trusts, most values centre on:

- Care and Compassion
- Respect and Dignity
- Integrity and Accountability
- Teamwork and Collaboration
- Quality and Excellence

This question tests whether you understand and live by those values in your daily professional practice.

You are expected to show that you:

- Understand what the Trust values mean in action, not just in words.
- Can relate your behaviour and decisions to these values in the lab.
- Demonstrate professionalism, respect, and commitment to patient safety and service quality.
- Appreciate that your conduct affects both the patient outcome and the reputation of the Trust.

Answer:

I make a conscious effort to reflect the Trust's values in my daily practice as a Biomedical Scientist.

Care and Compassion:

Even though we work behind the scenes, I always remember that every sample represents a patient waiting for answers. For example, **in Haematology**, when processing urgent samples from A&E, I ensure prompt analysis and communication of critical results, which is motivated by care and compassion and understanding of how my action could impact on patient management.

Respect and Dignity:

I treat all colleagues, from support staff to clinicians with respect and understanding. **In Microbiology,** for example, if a junior colleague struggles with a new culture technique, I take the time to guide them patiently, maintaining dignity and mutual respect.

Integrity and Accountability:

I take full responsibility for my work and adhere to SOPs and quality standards. **In Blood Transfusion,** if I detect a potential discrepancy in patient identification or crossmatch results, I will immediately halt the process, investigate, and escalate to ensure patient safety rather than taking shortcuts.

Teamwork and Collaboration:

Laboratory work relies heavily on collaboration. During busy on-call shifts, I coordinate effectively with colleagues across departments, for example, supporting Biochemistry during high sample loads while ensuring my own area runs smoothly.

Quality and Excellence:

I continuously look for ways to improve the service by attending CPD sessions, participating in audits, and contributing to non-conformance reviews. **In Histopathology**, I once suggested a checklist system for specimen reception that helped reduce sample mismatch incidents.

Summary:

I live out the Trust's values by treating colleagues with respect, taking accountability for my actions, showing compassion for patients, and striving for quality in everything I do. These values guide my professional behaviour and ensure that the service I deliver contributes positively to both patient outcomes and the wider reputation of the Trust.

Question 159:

When was your integrity questioned?

Background:

Integrity is one of the most important values in laboratory practice. It means being honest, transparent, and accountable for your actions, especially when something goes wrong. In the NHS and other accredited laboratories, integrity builds trust between staff, patients, and clinical users. This question tests your ability to handle situations where your professional honesty, judgement, or actions were questioned and how you responded in line with ethical and professional standards such as the HCPC Code of Conduct, ISO 15189, and Trust Values.

You are expected to show that you:

- Understand the importance of professionalism, honesty, integrity in laboratory work.
- Stay calm and factual when your integrity is questioned.
- Respond professionally and calmly when questioned or challenged.
- Use evidence, documentation, or audit trails to support your position.
- Value transparency and accountability over defensiveness.
- Take every situation as a learning experience to improve communication and trust.

Answer 1:

Integrity is essential in laboratory practice, where patient safety depends on the accuracy and reliability of our results.

A situation occurred early in my career when I was working **in Haematology**. A senior colleague questioned me because a result I validated appeared inconsistent with the previous sample for the same patient. I remained calm and explained my validation process, showing that I had followed the standard operating procedure (SOP), checked internal quality control (IQC), and confirmed the analyser flags before releasing the result.

To ensure transparency, I rechecked the sample with a colleague, reran the analysis, and confirmed that the result was accurate. The difference was due to the patient's clinical condition rather than an analytical error. This incident reinforced the importance of maintaining clear documentation and open communication with colleagues.

In another instance **in Blood Transfusion**, a clinician queried why a crossmatch result was delayed. Rather than becoming defensive, I calmly explained that there was a positive antibody screen, and additional identification was needed for safe transfusion. This demonstrated professional honesty and prioritising patient safety over speed, which strengthened trust between the laboratory and clinical team.

Answer 2:

Integrity is a key part of my professional identity as a Biomedical Scientist. There was a time **in Haematology** when my integrity was questioned after I released a result that was slightly outside the expected range for a known patient. A colleague queried why I validated the result without repeating the test. I calmly explained that the result was consistent with the patient's historical trend, and the analyser QC was within range. I showed the previous results on LIMS and my validation notes, which confirmed my reasoning was appropriate. After reviewing together, we both agreed the decision was valid. I also reflected that documenting reasoning behind such decisions clearly helps prevent misunderstanding.

In Blood Transfusion, my integrity was once questioned when a clinician queried why I rejected a blood sample for being haemolysed during a major haemorrhage. I explained that accepting a compromised sample could lead to incorrect crossmatching and risk patient safety. I followed MHRA and BSH guidelines, escalated the case to the senior BMS, and communicated the decision clearly to the ward. The clinician later appreciated that my action was in the patient's best interest, which reinforced my confidence in standing by professional and safety standards.

In Biochemistry, a similar situation occurred when a potassium result was questioned by a doctor who believed it was falsely high. I reviewed the sample and noticed it was haemolysed. I explained that red cell breakdown can release intracellular potassium, causing a false increase. I documented my findings, rejected the result, and requested a repeat sample. This transparency strengthened clinical trust and demonstrated professional integrity.

In Microbiology, my integrity was challenged when a colleague disagreed with my decision to report a culture as "no significant growth." I reviewed the culture plates with the senior scientist, and our discussion confirmed my interpretation was correct. I learned the importance of involving others objectively when differences arise. It promotes shared understanding and maintains trust within the team.

In Histopathology, integrity was demonstrated when a discrepancy occurred in slide labelling. I immediately stopped the process, checked the patient identifiers, and reported the incident to my manager. The error was traced back to a batch labelling issue, and my prompt reporting prevented a potential patient misidentification. Although it caused temporary workflow delays, it highlighted the importance of always prioritising accuracy and transparency over speed.

Summary 1:

When my integrity was questioned, I responded calmly, professionally, and with evidence of my actions. I used the opportunity to clarify my process, ensure transparency, and strengthen communication. Such experiences have reinforced my commitment to accuracy, honesty, and accountability, which are values that are essential to safe and effective laboratory practice.

Summary 2:

I have learnt that integrity means doing what is right even when it is uncomfortable or misunderstood. By being honest, following SOPs, documenting decisions, and communicating

clearly, I protect patient safety and maintain professional trust. Whether it's validating results in Haematology, rejecting samples in Transfusion or Biochemistry, or identifying discrepancies in Microbiology or Histopathology, acting with integrity builds reliability and respect in the laboratory team and ultimately improves patient outcomes.

Question 160:

What do you do to ensure equipment is fit for use?

Background:

In a biomedical laboratory, ensuring that equipment is fit for use is critical for generating accurate, reliable, and safe results. Faulty or poorly maintained equipment can lead to analytical errors, delayed results, and potential harm to patients. This question tests your understanding of equipment maintenance, quality assurance, and good laboratory practice (GLP) in accordance with ISO 15189 standards.

You are expected to show that you:

- Understand the processes for ensuring equipment readiness and performance.
- Know the importance of documentation, maintenance, and calibration.
- Follow quality control and preventive maintenance procedures.
- Report, troubleshoot, or escalate issues appropriately.
- Appreciate that ensuring fitness for use protects patient safety and laboratory reputation.

Answer:

To ensure laboratory equipment is fit for use, I follow a systematic process that starts before, during, and after each use.

Firstly, at the start of my shift, I check that all analysers have passed daily internal quality control (IQC) and any required calibrations have been performed successfully. I verify that maintenance logs are up to date and that any previous faults have been resolved before using the equipment. For example, **in Biochemistry**, I ensure the analyser's temperature, reagent levels, and calibration curves are within acceptable limits before running patient samples.

Secondly, I perform daily, weekly, and monthly maintenance as scheduled in the equipment's SOP. This includes checking tubing, cleaning probes, and ensuring waste containers are emptied and disinfected. I record all maintenance activities in the equipment logbook or LIMS for traceability.

If an issue arises, such as a failed QC or error code, I do not proceed with patient samples. I troubleshoot according to the manufacturer's guide and SOP. For example, rechecking reagents, performing a recalibration, or contacting the engineer if necessary. I also escalate unresolved issues to the senior BMS or section lead and clearly label the instrument as "out of use" to prevent accidental operation.

In Haematology, this could mean confirming that the analyser has passed background counts and running control materials at multiple levels before validating patient results.

In Blood Transfusion, I ensure centrifuges, refrigerators, and alarm systems have been checked and recorded as compliant under MHRA and UKAS requirements.

In Microbiology, daily checks on incubator temperatures, autoclave validation, and equipment sterility records are essential for ensuring reliable culture results.

Summary:

I ensure equipment is fit for use by following SOPs, performing regular QC and maintenance, documenting all checks, and escalating any faults promptly. These practices ensure reliable, accurate, and traceable results, prevent errors, and maintain compliance with ISO 15189 and MHRA

standards, which ultimately supports patient safety and laboratory efficiency.

Question 161:

What would you do when equipment breakdown?

Background:

Laboratory equipment plays a crucial role in generating accurate and timely patient results. When an analyser or key instrument breaks down, it can significantly impact workflow, turnaround times (TAT), and patient care. This question tests your ability to respond calmly and professionally to equipment failure, ensuring continuity of service, patient safety, and adherence to ISO 15189, manufacturer recommendations, and Trust policies.

You are expected to show that you:

- Understand how to recognise and report equipment breakdowns.
- Follow SOPs for troubleshooting, escalation, and documentation.
- Communicate effectively with colleagues, engineers, and clinical users.
- Ensure continuity of service through contingency plans.
- Use initiative while maintaining safety and quality standards.

Answer:

If an equipment breakdown occurs, my first step is to remain calm and ensure the issue is correctly identified and isolated to prevent further disruption or errors. I would then follow the laboratory's SOP for analyser or equipment malfunction, which typically includes basic troubleshooting, escalation, and documentation.

For example, **in Haematology**, if the full blood count analyser stops mid-run (stop working while in the middle of sample analysis), I would first check for simple issues such as blocked sample probes, reagent levels, or waste container overflow. If these checks do not resolve the issue, I would take the analyser out of service, record the incident in the analyser logbook and Q-Pulse, and escalate the matter to the senior BMS or duty manager. Meanwhile, I would transfer urgent samples to another available analyser or, if necessary, refer them to another site as per the business continuity plan to maintain service delivery.

In Blood Transfusion, if the blood grouping analyser or crossmatch system breaks down, I would immediately switch to manual testing following SOP and inform the senior staff. I would also contact the engineer or manufacturer for urgent repair and ensure all results from the faulty analyser are withheld or verified manually to prevent erroneous results. I will also communicate with clinical staff. This is vital and expected to inform the wards of potential delays during major haemorrhage protocols or other urgent/emergency scenarios.

In Biochemistry, if an analyser such as a Roche Cobas or Abbott Alinity fails, I would perform basic checks like reviewing system error logs, reagent placement, or water supply. If unresolved, I would move testing to the backup analyser and notify clinical areas of expected delays for urgent samples such as cardiac troponin or electrolytes. All incidents would be documented in the instrument downtime log, and maintenance records reviewed before reintroducing the analyser to use.

In Microbiology, if the automated blood culture system or MALDI-TOF goes offline, I would ensure manual backup procedures are initiated. For example, subculturing positive bottles manually and recording timepoints to ensure continuity of diagnostic work.

In Histopathology, if the tissue processor breaks down overnight, I would keep tissues refrigerated and inform the senior scientist or on-call engineer first thing in the morning. For urgent specimens, I may refer samples to a linked network laboratory if available. Preventing tissue degradation and documenting chain-of-custody will remain my priority, as that would ensure patient safety.

After the issue is resolved, I would perform QC checks or validation runs to confirm the analyser's performance before resuming patient testing. I would also reflect on the incident to identify preventive measures. For example, improved maintenance schedules, clearer user logs, or early-warning alerts.

Summary:

When equipment breaks down, I follow the principle of safety, communication, continuity, and documentation. By staying calm, following SOPs, using backup systems, and communicating effectively, I help ensure patient results are not compromised. Whether in Haematology, Blood Transfusion, Biochemistry, Microbiology, or Histopathology, my focus is always on maintaining quality, patient safety, and service continuity while learning from each incident to strengthen laboratory resilience.

Question 162:

Why did you apply for this job?

Background:

Interviewers use this question to assess your motivation, understanding of the role, and alignment with the organisation's values and goals. For biomedical scientists, it is also a chance to show enthusiasm for continuous development, teamwork, patient care, and quality service. A strong answer connects your skills, experience, and aspirations directly to what the Trust or laboratory offers.

You are expected to show that you:

- Understand the role and responsibilities of the post.
- Are motivated by professional growth and quality service.
- Can demonstrate how your skills and experience align with the Trust's goals.
- Appreciate the laboratory's contribution to patient care.
- Provide practical examples that show your suitability.

Answer:

I applied for this job because it aligns perfectly with my professional goals, my passion for quality patient care, and my desire to continue developing as a biomedical scientist within a structured and forward-thinking organisation like this Trust.

Having worked across several departments, including Haematology, Blood Transfusion, and Biochemistry, I have developed a strong foundation in laboratory analysis, quality assurance, and multidisciplinary teamwork. This post provides the opportunity to build on those skills while contributing to a laboratory that values accuracy, innovation, and patient-centred care.

I am particularly attracted to this Trust because of its commitment to ISO 15189 standards, its strong focus on staff training, and its integration of new technologies. For example, I read about the laboratory's recent implementation of advanced analysers and automation, which demonstrates a clear dedication to improving turnaround times and maintaining accuracy, values that I strongly share.

In my current role, I have been involved in EQA and IQC reviews, staff competency training, and continuous improvement initiatives. These experiences have reinforced the importance of consistency, teamwork, and proactive problem solving, all of which are essential qualities for this role.

For example, **in Haematology,** I worked with my team to introduce a daily analyser maintenance checklist that reduced unexpected downtime. **In Blood Transfusion**, I supported new staff with crossmatch training to ensure safe issue of blood components. **In Biochemistry**, I helped review validation data for new reagent lots before use. These practical experiences have prepared me to make a meaningful contribution here.

Ultimately, I applied because I see this role not just as a job, but as an opportunity to add value to the service, learn from an experienced team, and grow within a Trust known for high standards and patient-centred care.

Summary:

I applied for this job because it represents the next step in my professional growth, offering a chance to apply my laboratory experience while contributing to a high-quality, patient-focused service. The Trust's values of excellence, teamwork, and integrity reflect how I already work, and I am eager to bring my experience, enthusiasm, and commitment to support the laboratory's continued success.

Question 163:

Tell us about your experience.

Background:

This question allows you to summarise your career journey, focusing on relevant technical, analytical, and interpersonal skills. It is not just about listing previous roles. Interviewers want to understand what you have done, what you have learned, and how your experience prepares you for this role. A strong answer gives a structured overview across training, key responsibilities, and achievements.

You are expected to show that you:

- Have practical laboratory experience relevant to the role.
- Understand how your work supports patient diagnosis and treatment.
- Have developed professionally through continuous learning.
- Can demonstrate adaptability, teamwork, and initiative.
- Link your past experience to how it prepares you for the advertised post.

Answer:

I have developed a broad range of experience working in accredited laboratories across Haematology, Blood Transfusion, and Biochemistry, with exposure to Microbiology and Histopathology processes through multidisciplinary collaboration.

My career began during my IBMS registration portfolio training, where I gained experience in sample reception, analytical testing, and understanding quality control principles. After registration, I took on responsibilities that strengthened both my technical and professional skills.

In Haematology, I perform full blood counts, ESRs, reticulocyte counts, and blood film reviews, ensuring all results are validated and clinically correlated. I have used analysers such as the Sysmex XN series and IL ACL TOP for coagulation studies. I actively troubleshoot issues like sample clots or flags on the analyser, and I work closely with clinicians when urgent results, such as critical haemoglobin or platelet counts, are identified.

In Blood Transfusion, I manage antibody screening, crossmatching, and issue of blood components using systems such as Ortho Vision or Bio-Rad IH-1000 and LIMS respectively. I strictly adhere to MHRA and UKAS standards, ensuring traceability and patient safety. For example, I once supported the implementation of a new antibody screening reagent and contributed to the local validation and documentation process.

In Clinical Biochemistry, I operate and maintain automation such as Abbott Alinity c and Roche Cobas 8000. I ensure daily IQC checks are within range before releasing patient results, and I take part in EQA reviews to maintain consistency and accuracy.

I have also been involved in training and mentoring junior staff, assisting them in understanding practical bench work and documentation, which improved overall team confidence and performance.

Across all departments, I have been actively involved in Quality Management System (QMS) activities such as incident reporting, document reviews, and audits. Thereby, supporting continuous service improvement and regulatory compliance.

I am confident that my hands-on experience, technical knowledge, and commitment to maintaining high-quality laboratory standards have prepared me well for this role.

Summary:

My experience spans across major diagnostic disciplines, combining technical competence, problem-solving, and teamwork. I have learned the importance of accuracy, patient safety, and continuous learning in ensuring effective laboratory service delivery, which are values I will continue to uphold in this role.

Question 164:

When did you fail and what did you do.

Background:

This question is designed to assess self-awareness, accountability, and resilience. In laboratory practice, mistakes or setbacks may occur, but what matters most is how they are handled and what lessons are learned. Employers want to see that you can take responsibility, reflect, and use such experiences to improve performance and prevent recurrence.

You are expected to show that you:

- Can acknowledge and take ownership of your mistakes.
- Follow the correct reporting procedures (e.g., Datix, Q-pulse, or internal incident forms).
- Understand the importance of reflection and corrective action.
- Learn from the experience to prevent similar incidents.
- Maintain professionalism and protect patient safety.

Answer:

I believe failure is an opportunity to learn and improve. One example that stands out was during my early days **in Haematology** when I once missed a delta check flag on a full blood count result due to a busy workload. The analyser had indicated a sudden drop in haemoglobin compared to the patient's previous result. I released the result but shortly afterwards, on routine review, I noticed the flag and realised it should have been verified before authorisation.

I immediately informed my senior biomedical scientist, and together we reviewed the case. A repeat sample was requested, which confirmed that the initial sample had been partially clotted, causing a falsely low haemoglobin. I documented the incident through our QMS system, reflected on the cause, and later discussed it during a team debrief session. Since then, I have made it a habit to carefully review all flags and delta checks before result authorisation, regardless of workload pressure.

Similarly, **in Blood Transfusion**, I once entered an incorrect unit number during component issue but realised it before final authorisation. I cancelled the transaction immediately and rechecked with another colleague to verify. This reinforced my practice of always performing a second person check and slowing down during critical steps, especially when working under pressure.

In Microbiology, I once prepared a plate with an incorrect antibiotic disk. When it was spotted by a colleague during daily bench check, I was transparent, owned up, and we replaced the plate before incubation. The experience reminded me of the importance of double-checking materials during setup.

These experiences taught me that being honest and proactive after a mistake maintains both team trust and patient safety. It also strengthened my commitment to continuous improvement and adherence to quality procedures.

Summary:

Failure is part of professional growth. What defines a competent Biomedical Scientist is not the absence of mistakes but the ability to recognise, report, and learn from them. By staying accountable, reflective, and transparent, I

ensure continuous improvement and uphold the integrity of patient care.

Question 165:

How do you approach a busy day.

Background:

In a pathology laboratory, busy days are common due to increased sample volumes, staff shortages, urgent clinical requests, or equipment downtime. How a biomedical scientist approaches a busy day affects patient safety, turnaround time (TAT), and overall laboratory efficiency. This question is testing your organisational skills, ability to prioritise tasks, and resilience under pressure.

You are expected to show that you:

- Recognise factors that make a day busy and how to plan for them.
- Can prioritise tasks effectively to maintain patient care and TAT.
- Use practical examples to demonstrate organisation and decision-making.

Answer:

When I approach a busy day, I start by reviewing all pending tasks and identifying urgent or time-sensitive requests. I make a priority list, separating critical patient samples (e.g., emergency crossmatches, critical biochemistry results, or urgent microbiology cultures) from routine work. I ensure that equipment is functioning correctly, and if there are any known issues, I plan contingencies.

I also communicate with my team, where available, to delegate tasks appropriately and ensure that everyone is clear about their responsibilities. For example, in haematology, I would prioritise a critical A&E sample for a full blood count while routine inpatient samples are queued. In blood transfusion, I ensure that emergency crossmatches or MHP notifications are processed immediately, with less urgent routine blood requests managed thereafter. In microbiology, urgent cultures from suspected sepsis cases are processed ahead of routine screening samples. In histopathology, urgent intraoperative frozen sections are prioritised over routine biopsies.Throughout the day, I remain flexible, re-evaluating priorities as new samples arrive or if equipment issues arise. I also keep clear documentation and communicate with clinicians if delays are expected, ensuring transparency and patient safety.

Summary:

I approach a busy day by planning and prioritising effectively, maintaining patient safety and turnaround time. I balance urgent and routine work, remain flexible to changing circumstances, and communicate clearly with colleagues and clinicians. These demonstrate my ability to maintain high-quality service under pressure while ensuring that critical tasks are addressed first.

Question 166:

What do you do to ensure internal quality control in your laboratory.

Answer:

I ensure internal quality control (IQC) is maintained by following established SOPs and participating actively in daily quality assurance procedures.

Before running any patient samples, I make sure that the internal quality controls are analysed and within the acceptable target ranges defined by our laboratory's QC policy. I check both the Levey-Jennings charts and Westgard rules to identify any trends, shifts, or outliers that might indicate analytical issues.

If a control result falls outside the acceptable limits, I stop testing, quarantine the affected analyser or reagent batch, and begin troubleshooting. This includes checking reagent expiry dates, calibration status, sample integrity, and instrument maintenance logs. I then document all actions taken in accordance with ISO 15189 requirements and the lab's quality management system.

I also contribute to continuous quality improvement by reviewing QC data regularly with colleagues and the senior BMS to identify patterns and propose preventive actions. This ensures ongoing accuracy, reliability, and compliance with UKAS accreditation standards.

Ultimately, I see IQC not just as a tick-box exercise, but as a critical safeguard to ensure patient results are valid, traceable, and clinically reliable.

Question 167:

Choose one of our values that most suit yours

Answer:

Before applying for this role, I took time to look at the Trust's values, which are: Working together for patients, Respect and dignity, Commitment to quality of care, Compassion, improving lives, and Everyone counts.

The value that resonates most with me is 'Everyone counts.' I believe this value really underpins all the others, because providing high-quality, compassionate care relies on recognising the importance of every individual, which include both patients and staff.

In my work as a Biomedical Scientist, I see this through the way we treat every sample and every result with equal care and attention. Each one represents a patient who's relying on us for accurate answers. I make sure to follow SOPs, maintain quality standards, and support colleagues so that we can all contribute effectively to patient care.

I also think 'Everyone counts' extends to teamwork and inclusivity by respecting different skills, experiences, and perspectives within the lab helps us deliver the best possible service. So, for me, this value is not just about equality; it's about recognising that every person, and every role, is vital to achieving the Trust's overall commitment to quality and patient care.

Question 168:

Importance of quality control whilst running your samples and how to achieve it?

Answer:

Quality control is absolutely essential when running samples because it ensures that the results we release are accurate, reliable, and clinically valid. Every result we produce contributes to a patient's diagnosis or treatment plan, so maintaining strict quality control protects patient safety and upholds confidence in the laboratory service.

To achieve this, I make sure that internal quality control (IQC) is performed before analysing patient samples, using control materials with known target values. I check that results fall within the acceptable limits on Levey-Jennings charts and follow Westgard rules to detect any trends, shifts, or errors.

If controls are out of range, I stop patient testing immediately, investigate the cause such as reagent issues, instrument malfunction, or calibration drift and document all actions as part of the quality management system in line with ISO 15189 standards.

In addition to daily IQC, I also ensure that we participate in external quality assessment (EQA) schemes, which provide independent verification of our accuracy compared to other laboratories. Reviewing both IQC and EQA data helps identify areas for improvement and supports continuous quality assurance.

Ultimately, consistent and well-documented quality control gives clinicians confidence that the results they receive are trustworthy and that is central to safe, effective patient care.

Question 169:

How would you manage contamination after running laboratory test investigation and assuring that the right result is produced?

Answer:

If I suspected contamination after running a laboratory test, my first priority would be to ensure that no inaccurate results are reported. I would stop releasing any affected results immediately and quarantine the batch or instrument involved.

Next, I would review the QC data and repeat the internal quality control to determine whether the issue is isolated or widespread. I would then retest the affected samples, ideally using fresh reagents or a different analyser if available, to verify the accuracy of the results.

At the same time, I would carry out a root cause investigation by checking possible contamination sources such as reagents, consumables, pipettes, or environmental factors, and reviewing whether aseptic techniques or workflow practices were compromised.

All findings and corrective actions would be documented within the quality management system in line with ISO 15189 and UKAS requirements, and I would escalate the incident to the senior Biomedical Scientist or Quality Lead.

Once the issue is resolved and verified through repeat testing and acceptable QC performance, I would ensure only the validated, accurate results are authorised and released.

Finally, would take part in any review or staff discussion to identify preventive measures such as retraining, workflow changes, or enhanced cleaning protocols to minimise the risk of recurrence.

By following this structured approach, I make sure that patient safety and result integrity remain at the centre of everything we do in the laboratory.

Question 170:

How did you prepare for this interview and why do you think you are the best person for the job?

Answer:

In preparing for this interview, I made sure to familiarise myself with the Trust and the department to really understand what matters most here. I reviewed the Trust's values, which are: Working together for patients, Respect and dignity, Commitment to quality of care, Compassion, improving lives, and Everyone counts and thought carefully about how these align with my own professional principles and day-to-day practice.

I also read through the person specification and job description in detail, identifying the key requirements such as maintaining quality standards, following UKAS ISO 15189 procedures, working effectively as part of a multidisciplinary team, and contributing to continuous improvement. I reflected on examples from my own experience where I have demonstrated these skills, such as managing quality control, troubleshooting analyser issues, and supporting colleagues under pressure.

In addition, I researched the Trust's recent developments and priorities, such as [Please insert relevant example if you know it e.g. "implementing a new LIMS system," or "expanding specialist testing services"], to understand how I could contribute to those goals from day one.

As for why I believe I am the best person for the job: I bring not only the technical competence and attention to detail required for accurate, reliable results, but also a strong sense of teamwork, accountability, and patient focus. I am committed to continuous learning, maintaining high quality standards, and supporting the wider goals of the Trust.

I believe my combination of scientific knowledge, quality-driven approach, and alignment with the Trust's values makes me well-suited to contribute positively to the laboratory and to the care we ultimately provide to patients.

Haematology - Example Answer:

To prepare for this interview, I reviewed the Trust's values and the person specification carefully to understand the expectations for a Biomedical Scientist in Haematology. I also refreshed my knowledge on the key areas of the department including full blood counts, coagulation studies, and morphological review, as well as the importance of maintaining strict internal and external quality control in automated analysers and manual differentials.

I also read about recent developments in the Trust's pathology services, such as the implementation of digital morphology systems and automation lines.

I believe I am well-suited for this role because I have strong analytical skills, experience troubleshooting analyser errors, and a meticulous approach to reviewing abnormal blood films and authorising results. I work well under pressure, communicate effectively with clinicians when urgent results are needed, and always prioritise patient safety through accurate, timely reporting.

Blood Transfusion - Example Answer:

In preparation, I made sure to familiarise myself with the Trust's transfusion policies, MHRA and UKAS requirements, and the person specification for this post. I reviewed my knowledge of antibody screening, crossmatching, issue procedures, and the importance of traceability and documentation in accordance with BSQR and ISO 15189 standards.

I also looked at how the Trust promotes patient blood management and safety.

I believe I am the right candidate because I have a strong understanding of the critical importance of accuracy and haemovigilance in transfusion. I am confident using LIMS and blood tracking systems, responding to emergency requests calmly, and communicating clearly with clinical staff to ensure the right blood product reaches the right patient at the right time. My attention to detail and commitment to safety directly reflect the Trust's value of 'Commitment to quality of care.'

Clinical Biochemistry - Example Answer:

To prepare for this interview, I reviewed the person specification, Trust values, and the department's role in delivering high-quality biochemical analyses to support patient care. I also refreshed my knowledge of key analytical platforms, such as Roche or Abbott analysers, calibration procedures, and the use of Levey-Jennings charts and Westgard rules for internal quality control.

I familiarised myself with the Trust's priorities, such as reducing turnaround times and maintaining UKAS accreditation.

I am confident that I am well-suited to this position because I have experience in routine and specialist biochemistry testing. I can identify and troubleshoot analytical errors effectively and always ensure QC results are within range before authorising patient results. I am also committed to continuous improvement and collaborative working values that align closely with the Trust's commitment to quality care and teamwork.

Microbiology - Example Answer:

In preparing for this interview, I studied the person specification carefully and reviewed my knowledge of the core areas of microbiology such as biological sample culture, sensitivity testing, molecular diagnostics, and infection control. I also looked at the Trust's involvement in antimicrobial stewardship and infection prevention, as these are key priorities across NHS microbiology labs.

I also reviewed ISO 15189 standards for contamination control and quality assurance in microbiology testing.

I believe I am a strong fit because I have experience identifying and confirming clinically significant organisms, performing susceptibility testing accurately, and communicating urgent results effectively to clinical teams. I am meticulous about maintaining aseptic technique and documentation, and I understand the impact our results have on patient management and public health.

Histopathology - Example Answer:

Before this interview, I reviewed the Trust's values, the person specification, and the standards required for high-quality diagnostic histopathology. I also refreshed my knowledge of tissue processing, embedding, microtomy, and staining protocols, as well as quality control procedures that ensure slide integrity and staining consistency.

I read about how the Trust is working towards digital pathology and automation, which I find exciting as it enhances efficiency and diagnostic accuracy.

I believe I am the right person for this role because I am meticulous, organised, and committed to maintaining quality at every stage of the histology process. I take pride in producing slides that enable clear, accurate reporting by pathologists, and I always follow SOPs carefully to maintain safety, traceability, and consistency. My attention to detail and quality focus directly reflects the Trust's values of 'Commitment to quality of care' and 'Everyone counts.

Question 171:

Tell me what you know about the trust and trust values

Answer:

Before applying for this role, I made sure to research the Trust to understand its mission, priorities, and core values. I know the Trust is committed to delivering high-quality, patient-centred care across a range of acute and specialist services, and it emphasises teamwork, innovation, and continuous improvement. These principles align closely with my own approach to laboratory work.

The Trust's values are Working together for patients, Respect and dignity, Commitment to quality of care, Compassion, improving lives, and Everyone counts. I see these values as central to everything we do in the laboratory. For example, even though we work behind the scenes, every sample represents a person who is depending on us for accurate and timely results.

I have demonstrated the Trust values in my previous role as a biomedical scientist. For example:

- **Working together for patients:** In my previous role, I collaborated closely with clinicians and nurses to prioritise urgent samples for patients in A&E and ITU. By communicating clearly and working as a team, we helped ensure rapid turnaround times for critical tests like blood gases and coagulation screens.

- **Respect and dignity:** I treat every colleague and every sample with the same level of respect. For example, during busy periods, I always maintain professionalism, listen to others' viewpoints, and support junior staff who might be under pressure, which I believe help in creating a positive, respectful lab environment.

- **Commitment to quality of care:** Quality is at the heart of my work. I always review internal QC and EQA data carefully and once identified a drift in QC results. I usually investigate the primary root cause and that may led to recalibration and as a result prevent erroneous patient results being released. That experience reinforced for me how vital quality control is in maintaining safe, reliable care.

- **Compassion and improving lives:** I remind myself that each result I authorise represents someone's diagnosis, treatment, or reassurance. For example, when processing oncology or neonatal samples, I stay mindful that accuracy and timeliness can directly improve someone's life or reduce anxiety for a family.

- **Everyone counts:** I believe everyone in the lab contribution to patient care. I do my best to supported colleagues by taking on extra shifts, helping with training, and sharing good practice. Also, ensuring that the workload is fair and that we deliver consistent service quality across the team."

Overall, I feel my professional approach naturally reflects the Trust's values. I am excited about being motivated by accuracy, teamwork, and continuous improvement and I look forward to the opportunity, to contribute to a Trust that shares those same principles.

Question 172:

How would you handle a spillage?

Answer:

If a spillage occurred in the laboratory, my first priority would be to ensure everyone's safety. I would immediately stop what I am doing, alert colleagues nearby, and cordon off or clearly mark the area using caution slippery surface sign to prevent anyone entering until it is made safe.

Next, I would assess the type of spillage. For example, whether it is biological material such as blood, urine, or CSF, or a chemical reagent and then follow the appropriate COSHH and laboratory SOP guidance.

For example, I would wear the appropriate PPE such as lab coat, gloves, and eye protection and use the designated spillage kit. In our lab, that involves applying Chemgen, a chlorine-based disinfectant granule, directly onto the spill such as biological material. Chemgen effectively disinfects biological materials such as blood and body fluids. I would allow the recommended contact time, which is usually between 10 -15 minutes. That is to ensure complete disinfection before carefully wiping the area with absorbent material and disposing of all waste in the appropriate biohazard bags yellow bin. Also, ensure that sharp objects are placed in the sharp bin.

Once the area is clean and decontaminated, I would remove my PPE safely, wash my hands thoroughly, and document the incident according to SOP. I would also report the incident to the senior Biomedical Scientist or Health and Safety Officer, and if required, log it formally on Datix so that any lessons learned can be shared across the team.

If the spill involved a chemical or reagent instead, I would refer to the COSHH data sheet for that substance and follow the specific neutralisation and disposal instructions provided.

Overall, I would handle a spillage by keeping calm, acting quickly, using the right PPE and disinfectant (such as Chemgen), and following the Trust's safety procedures to ensure the area is properly disinfected and that there's no risk to staff or contamination of samples.

Question 173:

What would you do if there's an equipment downtime and where do you think equipment logs are kept?

Answer:

If an analyser or piece of laboratory equipment went down during testing, my first priority would be to stop using it immediately and make sure no further samples are processed until the issue is resolved. As patient safety and result reliability always come first.

I would then clearly label the analyser as 'out of service' to prevent accidental use and inform the senior Biomedical Scientist or duty manager right away where applicable. Next, I would check whether the issue can be resolved through basic troubleshooting. For example, checking power supply, reagent levels, or any error messages but only within the scope of what's allowed in the SOP.

If it is a significant fault that requires technical support, I would record all relevant details, including the time of failure, a description of the fault, and any troubleshooting carried out, in the equipment logbook. These records are usually kept either beside the instrument, in the equipment maintenance folder, or electronically on the laboratory's Quality Management System such as Q-Pulse. This ensures full traceability of faults, maintenance, and service history in line with ISO 15189 and UKAS accreditation requirements.

I would then follow the department's contingency plan. For example, switching to an alternative analyser, transferring testing to another site within the network, or prioritising urgent samples manually, depending on the test area. All affected samples would be documented and results clearly marked to indicate any delays on LIMS.

Once the engineer has resolved the issue, I would ensure that all relevant quality checks, calibrations, and internal quality controls are performed before the analyser is put back into service. Only once QC performance is verified would I resume patient testing.

By following these steps such as isolating the equipment, documenting everything in the equipment log, escalating promptly, and verifying performance before use, I can ensure that quality, traceability, and patient safety are maintained throughout the downtime

Question 174:

What is a hazard and what is a risk?

Answer:

A hazard is anything that has the potential to cause harm, damage, or adverse effect on health. For example, a biological agent such as blood or bacteria, a chemical reagent, sharp instrument, or even faulty equipment has a potential to cause harm, damage to individuals, leading adverse effect on the person health.

A risk, on the other hand, is the likelihood that the hazard will actually cause harm, and how severe that harm could be.

We can say that the hazard is the danger itself, while the risk is the chance of that danger causing injury, infection, or damage.

For example, in a haematology or microbiology lab, blood samples are a hazard because they could contain infectious agents like hepatitis or HIV. The risk then depends on how likely it is that someone could be exposed to the hazard. For example, not wearing a PPE or PPE not worn properly can expose a biomedical scientist or other pathology staff members to infectious agent or if a sharps injury occurs, leading to adverse effect on health. However, by using gloves, lab coats, and following safe disposal procedures, we reduce the risk of that hazard causing harm.

That is why risk assessments are carried out in the lab. The aim is to identify hazards, evaluate the risks, and put control measures in place to keep staff and patients safe in line with COSHH regulations.

Question 175:

How have you carried out supervision and management duties in current job

Answer:

In my previous and current role, I have been responsible for both supervisory and management day to day duties. This have helped to learned how to balance each of these tasks effectively depending on the demands of the laboratory. For example, on a typical day, I supervise staff at the bench, ensuring they follow SOPs, perform IQC correctly, and maintain accurate documentation. At the same time, I manage key administrative and quality tasks such as signing off competencies, reviewing EQA and QC reports, attending departmental meetings, and investigating any non-conformances or incidents.

To complete the task effectively - I prioritise the tasks based on assessing what is most critical for patient safety and service continuity at any given time. For example, if a staff member needs immediate training support on an analyser or a competency review, I give that my attention because it directly impacts testing accuracy and staff confidence. Once that is stabilised, I return to my management tasks like updating QC summaries, writing up incident investigations, or preparing reports for quality meetings.

I also use good time management and communication to keep things running smoothly. For example, delegating certain routine checks or documentation to competent staff, so I can focus on higher-level tasks when needed. Flexibility is also a key for me. For example, some days require more hands-on bench supervision, while others are better suited for administrative work such as reviewing training records or preparing for audits.

Overall, I maintain a clear focus on quality and patient safety while supporting staff development. I see both supervision and management as part of the same goal, ensuring a safe, efficient, and continuously improving laboratory service.

For example, during a recent EQA review, I identified a pattern that required staff retraining. I scheduled a short session at the start of the shift, so it didn't disrupt workflow. I then documented the competency updates and later completed the EQA summary for the quality meeting. That experience showed me the importance of being flexible and using time efficiently to manage both people and quality responsibilities.

Question 176:

Tell us ways in which you have managed conflict in the course of your duties

Answer:

In any laboratory environment, where work can be fast-paced and pressures are high, occasional conflict can occur. This can be due to difference in opinion, communication misunderstanding, or workload tension. In my role, I have learned to approach such situations calmly, objectively, and with respect for everyone involved.

One example was when two colleagues disagreed over prioritising urgent samples during a busy on-call shift. Rather than allowing the disagreement to escalate, I stepped in as the supervising BMS and asked both staff to pause and explain their viewpoints. I acknowledged their concerns and referred back to our departmental SOP and Trust escalation policy, which clearly outline how urgent samples should be managed. Once everyone understood the agreed process, we redistributed the workload so that both routine and urgent samples were handled safely. After the shift, I spoke to each person individually to check in and then raised the issue briefly at the next team huddle as a learning point. Focusing on communication and teamwork rather than blame.

By staying neutral, listening actively, and using policy as a guide, I was able to resolve the conflict quickly and maintain service continuity. I also reminded the team that our common goal is patient safety, which helped refocus everyone's perspective.

I believe managing conflict effectively is about maintaining respect and dignity, keeping communication open, and resolving issues early before they affect quality or morale. Also, at the end it can act as a learning curve and team improvement.

Question 177:

Have you been involved in developing a new method or equipment? Tell us how you did it

Answer:

Yes, I have been involved in developing and validating new methods in the laboratory. One example was when our department introduced a new analyser for [insert your discipline e.g., biochemistry or haematology], which required validation before it could be used for routine patient testing.

I was part of the project team responsible for implementing the method. My role included:

- Reviewing manufacturer guidance and SOPs to understand the correct operating procedures and limitations of the analyser.

- Planning and performing method verification studies, which included running parallel tests with the existing analyser, checking linearity, precision, accuracy, and comparing results using quality control materials and patient samples.

- Documenting all procedures and results in line with ISO 15189 requirements to ensure full traceability.

- Analysing data to identify any trends, biases, or discrepancies, and discussing findings with senior staff and the multidisciplinary team.

- Training colleagues on the new method once it was validated, including demonstrating SOPs, competency checks, and troubleshooting guidance.

By following a structured approach, we were able to validate the new analyser safely and efficiently. It improved turnaround times for our routine tests, reduced manual errors, and maintained compliance with UKAS and Trust quality standards.

Question 178:

What approach will you take to teaching a younger colleague?

Answer:

When teaching or mentoring a younger colleague, my approach is supportive, structured, and patient-centred. Firstly, I always start by understanding the current level of knowledge and experience of the colleague. For example, whether they are a trainee, new starter, or student on placement. That helps me tailor the training to their needs to become competent and able to carry any given task inline with their scope of practice.

I like to use a **'show, explain, do'** method: first I demonstrate the correct technique according to the SOP, then explain why each step is important in relation to quality and patient safety, and finally supervise them while they carry it out themselves. I encourage questions at every stage and provide constructive feedback immediately, focusing on what went well and where improvement is needed.

I also make sure all training is properly documented on the competency matrix or training record, in line with ISO 15189 requirements. Once the colleague **has** gained confidence, I gradually increase their independence while still reviewing their work until they are fully competent.

For example, when training a junior colleague on operating the haematology analyser, I first demonstrated the daily maintenance and QC procedures, then supervised them performing it for several days. We can review QC trends together, so that the colleague can be able to understand what to look for, and once knowledge of what to expect has been consistently demonstrated, I then signed off their competency. This not only built their confidence but ensured quality results for patients. This may vary slightly with a colleague with previous experience. I may have to firstly determine how previous experience is consistent with our Trust. That would allow me focus on what we do and if confidence and understanding is established. I then signed off competency.

Overall, my approach is respectful, patient, and focused on developing both technical skill and professional confidence. I see teaching as part of maintaining quality and supporting the next generation of Biomedical Scientists in delivering safe, effective care.

Question 179:

What are the different training methods you use in your current role?

Answer:

In my current role, I use a variety of training methods depending on the complexity of the task, the trainee's experience level, and the learning outcomes required. My main goal is always to ensure the colleague becomes confident, competent, and safe to work independently in line with SOPs and ISO 15189 standards.

Some of the key training methods I use include:

Demonstration and Observation:

I begin by demonstrating the correct technique or procedure myself, step by step, while explaining the rationale behind each stage. For example, why specific QC checks or pipetting techniques are essential for accuracy. The trainee then repeats the process under supervision while I observe and provide feedback.

Guided Practice and Supervised Hands-on Training:

Once they have seen the procedure, I let them perform it independently under supervision. I encourage them to talk through what they are doing so I can assess both practical skills and understanding. This method works well for technical tasks like analyser maintenance or sample processing.

One-to-One Mentoring and Reflective Discussion:

I use informal discussions to reflect on learning experiences. For example, asking what went well and what could be improved. This builds critical thinking and confidence, particularly for problem-solving or troubleshooting situations.

Use of Training Documentation and Competency Frameworks:

All training is supported by written SOPs, training records, and competency checklists. I make sure trainees understand how to use these documents to guide their learning and ensure traceability for audits. For example, referring trainees to the SOPs for a given task to be train on before the training commencement.

E-learning and Structured Tutorials:

For theoretical topics such as health and safety, COSHH, or quality management, I direct staff to e-learning modules or short presentations, followed by practical sessions to link theory with practice.

Peer Learning and Shadowing:

I sometimes pair new staff with experienced colleagues so they can learn different techniques and gain confidence through observation and peer support.

For example, when training a colleague on blood transfusion analyser use, I started with a demonstration, followed by supervised practice. Then, we reviewed their results together using a reflective discussion to reinforce understanding before completing their competency sign-off. This structured approach ensures both learning and quality are maintained.

By combining these approaches, I am able to accommodate different learning styles such as visual, auditory, and hands-on, and that ensure consistent standards across the team. I also regularly review progress and provide constructive feedback until the trainee is fully competent and confident.

Question 180:

When your computer system goes down, what do you do and how does it affect turnaround time?

Answer:

If the computer or LIMS system goes down during testing, my first step would be to remain calm and follow the laboratory's contingency plan for IT or network failure. I would immediately inform the senior Biomedical Scientist or duty manager and the IT department so they can begin resolving the issue."

In the meantime, I would switch to manual or semi-manual processes as per the SOP. For example, we would continue to process samples on the analysers, but record patient details, sample numbers, and results manually on downtime worksheets or printouts. This ensures full traceability of all work carried out during the downtime.

Once the system is restored, I would carefully enter or verify all manually recorded results into LIMS, ensuring that the correct patient details are matched and double-checked by a second staff member to avoid transcription errors.

A system downtime will inevitably affect turnaround times to some extent, particularly in high-volume areas such as Haematology or Biochemistry. However, by prioritising urgent and critical samples, such as those from ITU or A&E, and maintaining clear communication with clinical staff about expected delays, we can minimise the impact on patient care.

All actions taken would be documented in the downtime log, including the time of system failure, the duration, and any samples processed manually. Once normal operations resume, I would participate in reviewing the incident and suggesting improvements for future downtime resilience.

In summary, while computer downtime can delay routine work slightly, following the contingency plan, maintaining traceability, and prioritising urgent samples ensures patient care remains unaffected and results remain reliable.

Examples - Haematology / Biochemistry:

During a LIMS outage, we continued analyser runs and manually recorded urgent results, phoning critical values directly to wards to prevent treatment delays.

Examples - Microbiology:

We logged specimens manually in a downtime book and used paper worksheets for culture and sensitivity reporting, then verified results electronically once the system was restored.

Examples - Blood Transfusion:

If the transfusion LIMS is unavailable, we revert to manual compatibility testing and handwritten traceability labels in accordance with the MHRA and SHOT guidelines, ensuring every step is double-checked by two staff before any issue of blood.

Question 181:

If you have any reason to go back to using manual methods for your work, how will it affect the staff strength and what will you do?

Answer:

If we had to revert to manual methods - for example, due to analyser failure, power outage, or LIMS downtime. it would naturally place more pressure on staff because manual processing is slower, more labour-intensive, and requires additional verification steps to maintain accuracy. It could therefore affect turnaround times and the number of samples we can process with the same staff strength.

In such a situation, my first action would be to assess the workload and staffing levels available, then prioritise testing based on clinical urgency. For example, A&E, ITU, and transfusion requests would come first. I would communicate with the senior BMS or section lead, to agree on a temporary workflow plan."

If necessary, I would reassign staff from less critical tasks to support manual work, ensuring each person is trained and competent in the relevant procedures. Teamwork and communication become even more important in these situations, so I would hold a brief huddle to ensure everyone understands their role, the priorities, and the safety checks required.

I would also inform clinical areas of the situation, so they are aware of possible delays, and document all actions taken. Once the issue is resolved and automated systems are back online, we would double-check all manually processed results before releasing them electronically.

While reverting to manual methods can temporarily affect efficiency, having a well-coordinated team, clear communication, and adherence to SOPs ensures we continue to provide a safe and reliable service for patients.

For example, during a short analyser breakdown in Haematology, we switched to manual differential counts and manual haemoglobin estimation. This required more time per sample, so I reassigned two staff from the morphology bench to support the urgent workload while routine samples were temporarily delayed. Once the analyser was back online, we verified and entered all results, maintaining full traceability.

Question 182:

Tell us about any health and safety incident you have encountered in the course of your job.

Answer:

In a laboratory environment, health and safety is a top priority, and I have experienced incidents that have reinforced the importance of following procedures carefully.

For example, during my time in [X department, e.g. Haematology], a colleague accidentally spilled a small amount of blood sample on the workbench while loading specimens onto the analyser. I immediately stopped what I was doing, helped to contain the spill, and ensured the area was cordoned off. We followed the department's spillage SOP, wearing appropriate PPE and using Chemgen disinfectant granules to decontaminate the area. Once the contact time had elapsed, the area was cleaned and all waste disposed of as biohazard.

We then documented the incident on Datix and informed the senior Biomedical Scientist and Health and Safety Officer. A short review was carried out later that day to identify the cause. In this case, overfilled sample tubes were discovered as the primary root cause. That allows the opportunity to then reinforce good sample handling practice during handover. As a result, we implemented a refresher briefing on safe specimen loading and handling.

The incident was managed safely, no one was harmed, and it served as a useful reminder of the importance of vigilance, communication, and following safety protocols. I always make sure to report any near-misses or incidents, because every event is an opportunity to improve safety culture and prevent recurrence.

Example - Blood Transfusion:

During crossmatching, a small breakage occurred when a sample tube cracked inside the centrifuge. I stopped the run immediately, isolated the centrifuge, and followed the chemical and biological spill SOP to clean and disinfect the centrifuge and area. The incident was logged on Datix, and we later reviewed sample handling techniques and tube inspection procedures during training.

Example - Microbiology:

A spillage occurred while streaking a high-risk specimen. The area was immediately decontaminated using Chemgen, and the incident led to a review of how high-risk samples were labelled and handled in the processing area.

Example - Histopathology:

A small formalin spill occurred when transferring tissue cassettes. We evacuated the area, used the chemical spillage kit to clean and disinfect the area. The storage and transfer protocols was then reviewed afterwards.

Question 183:

Why do you want to leave your job to work with us?

Answer:

I have really enjoyed my time in my current role and have gained valuable experience across [X area, e.g. haematology and blood transfusion]. It has been a great foundation, but I now feel ready to progress to the next stage of my career in a setting that offers broader exposure, more complex cases, and greater opportunities for learning and development.

I was particularly attracted to this role within your Trust because it is a larger, busier laboratory that supports a wider range of specialised and routine investigations. I believe this environment will help me to expand my technical and analytical skills, while also giving me the opportunity to work alongside a multidisciplinary team and learn from experienced colleagues.

I have also looked into your Trust values, which are: Commitment to Quality of Care and Improving Lives, and these resonate strongly with me. This is because I take pride in ensuring that the results I produce are accurate and timely because they directly impact patient care.

Another factor for me is career progression. Your Trust has a strong record of supporting staff through training, CPD, and IBMS portfolio development, which aligns with my goal to advance my practice and take on greater responsibilities in the future.

On a practical note, your hospital is also closer to where I live, which means I can maintain a better work-life balance while still contributing fully to the team. Overall, I see this position as an opportunity to continue growing within a supportive and high-performing laboratory, where I can make a meaningful contribution to patient services.

Question 184:

What are your salary requirements?

Answer:

As this role is within the NHS, I understand that the salary is based on the Agenda for Change pay scales. So, I am happy to accept the appropriate salary for the band and point that reflects my skills, experience, and qualifications.

For me, the main motivation is the opportunity to develop my career in a supportive and progressive Trust, contribute to service improvement, and gain further experience in [X area of specialty -

e.g. haematology and transfusion]. I am confident that the salary associated with this band is fair and aligns with my expectations.

Question 185:

Do you think you are overqualified for this position?

Answer:

I would not say that I am overqualified. Rather, I believe my experience allows me to contribute effectively from day one and add value to the team. Every laboratory and Trust has its own systems, standards, and ways of working, and I see this as an opportunity to continue learning and developing while bringing my knowledge to support service quality.

I am aware that this role is a [Band X] position, and I fully understand and respect the expectations at this level. What is important to me is being in a role that allows me to deliver high-quality work, support my colleagues, and continue progressing within a well-structured and supportive Trust.

In fact, I believe my experience will help in mentoring junior staff, assisting with training, and ensuring that quality and safety standards are consistently met. So rather than being overqualified, I see myself as well-prepared and committed to contributing positively to this role.

Question 186:

Explain what GLP is and explain why GLP is followed in the lab.

Answer:

GLP stands for Good Laboratory Practice. It is a set of principles designed to ensure the quality, integrity, and reliability of laboratory work, covering everything from sample collection, testing, and recording, to reporting and archiving results. Essentially, GLP provides a framework that ensures all laboratory activities are carried out in a consistent, traceable, and safe manner.

In the NHS laboratory setting, following GLP is crucial because our results directly impact patient diagnosis and treatment. By adhering to GLP, we ensure that every step of the testing process from pre-analytical to post-analytical is controlled, documented, and auditable.

It also supports compliance with ISO 15189 and UKAS accreditation standards, which require laboratories to demonstrate consistent quality management and technical competence. Following GLP means that: equipment is regularly maintained and calibrated; reagents are within expiry date; staff are properly trained and competent; and all results can be traced back to the analyst, instrument, and reagent batch used.

Ultimately, GLP helps prevent errors, ensures reproducibility, and builds confidence in the validity of laboratory results. It protects both the patient and the laboratory by maintaining high professional and scientific standards.

For example (Note the examples given here can be applicable to any of the departments – below is just a guide), **in Haematology,** GLP ensures that analysers are checked daily using IQC, maintenance logs are completed, and abnormal results are reviewed and authorised appropriately. **In Transfusion**, GLP ensures all processes from sample labelling to issue of blood are fully traceable and double-checked, which is critical for patient safety and MHRA compliance. **In Biochemistry**, GLP ensures reagents are properly stored, calibration is verified, and results are validated before release. **In Microbiology,** GLP ensures that samples are handled in accordance with biosafety levels, contamination is avoided, and all results are accurately recorded and traceable. **In Histopathology,** GLP ensures accurate specimen tracking, correct tissue processing, and traceable slide preparation to maintain diagnostic accuracy.

Question 187:

Define SOP and what is the most important thing about a SOP

Answer:

SOP stands for Standard Operating Procedure. It is a written, step-by-step instruction designed to ensure that a specific laboratory task or process is carried out consistently, accurately, and safely by all staff.

The most important thing about an SOP is that it ensures consistency and reliability of results. Following SOPs guarantees that every analyst performs the procedure in the same way, using the same equipment, reagents, and techniques. This is essential for maintaining patient safety, data integrity, and compliance with regulatory standards such as ISO 15189 and UKAS.

Other key aspects of a good SOP include clarity, accessibility, and regular review. Staff should be trained in the SOP, and any updates must be communicated. It is also vital to document adherence to the SOP. For example, by signing logs or recording QC data, so that results are traceable and auditable. **In Haematology**, SOPs for FBC analyser operation ensure QC is checked daily, abnormal results are flagged, and morphology slides are prepared consistently. **In Blood Transfusion**, SOPs guarantee that crossmatching, blood issue, and sample labelling follow strict traceability rules to prevent errors. **In Biochemistry,** SOPs standardise analyser calibration, reagent handling, and result verification to maintain accuracy across all samples. **In Microbiology,** SOPs ensure safe handling of infectious specimens, culture techniques, and susceptibility testing are performed correctly. **In Histopathology**, SOPs standardise tissue processing, embedding, and staining so slides are reproducible and diagnostically reliable.

Question 188:

What is the purpose of Quality Manual?

Answer:

A Quality Manual is a key document within the laboratory's quality management system (QMS). Its main purpose is to describe how the laboratory meets the requirements of accreditation standards, such as ISO 15189, and how it ensures the quality, reliability, and safety of its services.

It outlines the laboratory's policies, procedures, and organisational structure, and sets out the responsibilities of staff in maintaining quality. Essentially, it provides a central reference that defines the scope of the laboratory's services, the processes for sample handling, testing, documentation, and reporting, as well as how the laboratory monitors and improves its performance.

The Quality Manual is important because it ensures that all staff work consistently, procedures are standardised, and there are traceability and accountability for all work. It also supports audits, inspections, and continuous improvement, helping the laboratory maintain accreditation and, most importantly, deliver safe and accurate results for patients.

Example - Haematology:

The Quality Manual outlines policies for analyser QC, morphology review, and result authorisation, ensuring all staff follow the same standards.

Example - Blood Transfusion:

It details traceability requirements, compatibility checks, and emergency procedures, critical for patient safety.

Example - Biochemistry:

It defines how daily calibrations, QC, and EQA participation are documented and monitored.

Example - Microbiology:

It specifies safe handling of pathogens, culture and susceptibility testing protocols, and how contamination or deviations are reported.

Example - Histopathology:

It sets out specimen handling, tissue processing, slide preparation, and reporting procedures, maintaining diagnostic consistency.

Question 189:

What are the main areas that UKAS examines during accreditation?

Answer:

UKAS examines all aspects of the laboratory service to make sure we meet ISO 15189 standards for quality and competence. Their assessment focuses on eight main areas that cover the entire testing pathway.

First is the Quality Management System, which includes policies, document control, audits, and continual improvement. Then they look at staff. For example, ensuring or determine that everyone is trained, competent, and working within their scope of practice.

The environment, equipment, and IT systems are also assessed to make sure conditions are suitable. For example, instruments are maintained and calibrated, and records are traceable. UKAS then examines the full testing cycle, which are from the pre-examination phase (like sample receipt and identification), the examination phase (the analytical process itself), and the post-examination phase (reviewing and releasing results).

Finally, they assess evaluation and quality assurance, which includes IQC, EQA, audits, and management review. It helps the UKAS to confirm that the lab monitors its own performance and continuously improves.

Altogether, these areas ensure that the laboratory is technically competent, consistently produces accurate and reliable results, and ultimately provides a safe and effective service for patients.

Question 190:

In your opinion, what are the most important aspects of laboratory work?

Answer:

In my opinion, the most important aspects of laboratory work are accuracy, quality, and patient safety. Every sample we handle represents a patient waiting for results that could influence critical clinical decisions. So, maintaining accuracy and reliability in everything we do is essential.

Quality assurance underpins this. For example, from following SOPs, running internal and external quality controls, to ensuring equipment is well maintained and calibrated. Adhering to good laboratory practice and UKAS ISO15189 standards ensures that our results are consistent and traceable.

Teamwork and communication are also key. The laboratory relies on good collaboration between biomedical scientists, clinicians, and other healthcare staff to ensure timely and appropriate testing.

Finally, continuous learning and professional development are important. For example, keeping up to date with new methods, technologies, and quality standards helps maintain a high level of competence and supports continual improvement in patient care.

Question 191:

What are the requirements of a document control system, and why is it important to control documents in the laboratory?

Answer:

A document control system is a key part of the laboratory's Quality Management System, as required by ISO 15189. It ensures that all laboratory documents such as SOPs, policies, forms, and work instructions are current, authorised, and used consistently by all staff.

The main requirements of a document control system include proper version control, clear approval and authorisation by senior staff, controlled distribution so everyone is using the most recent version, and the withdrawal or archiving of obsolete documents. All documents should be traceable, reviewed regularly, and accessible to staff when needed.

Controlling documents is essential because it prevents errors caused by outdated or incorrect procedures. It ensures consistency, standardisation, and compliance with accreditation requirements. It also supports training and competency assessment, since staff rely on SOPs and quality records to perform their duties correctly.

Ultimately, good document control protects patient safety by ensuring that every test and process in the lab is performed to the same validated and approved standard.

For example, **in Haematology**, if an analyser SOP was updated after a reagent change, the document control system ensures only the latest version is available to staff. Old copies are withdrawn immediately to prevent outdated instructions being followed.

Question 192:

What kind of information a controlled document must have?

Answer:

A controlled document must contain clear and traceable information that allows staff to identify, verify, and use the document correctly. This includes details such as the document title, unique identification number, version or revision number, date of issue, author, approver, and review date.

It should also state its purpose or scope, references to related documents or standards, and any procedures or instructions to be followed. A controlled document should show evidence of authorisation. For example, a signature or electronic approval to confirm it has been reviewed and approved for use.

Including this information ensures that staff are always working from the correct, approved version, supports traceability during audits or UKAS assessments, and maintains consistency across the laboratory.

For example, **in Blood Transfusion**, an SOP for crossmatching will have a document code, version number, author and approver names, and review date. When it is updated, the new version replaces the old one immediately, ensuring staff follow the most current validated process.

Question 193:

Tell me about Document Control and Q-Pulse

Answer:

Document control is a key part of the laboratory's Quality Management System, ensuring that all documents such as SOPs, forms, policies, and records are current, authorised, and used consistently by all staff. It is a requirement of ISO 15189 and helps maintain standardisation, traceability, and compliance across the lab.

The aim is to make sure everyone is working from the correct and approved version of a document. This involves version control, authorisation by senior staff, controlled distribution, and withdrawal of obsolete versions.

In our Trust, we use Q-Pulse, which is an electronic quality management software that manages document control digitally. Q-Pulse allows documents to be created, reviewed, approved, and distributed electronically, with automatic version tracking and audit trails. Staff can easily access the latest approved versions, and the system automatically flags documents due for review or those awaiting approval.

Q-Pulse also helps with other aspects of quality management such as recording incidents, audits, non-conformances, and staff training records. So, it integrates document control within the wider quality framework.

Overall, using Q-Pulse ensures that our laboratory maintains compliance with ISO 15189 and UKAS requirements, supports traceability, and helps provide a safe, consistent, and high-quality service for patients.

For example, when an SOP **in Haematology** is updated. Let say for a new analyser or reagent, the revised document is uploaded to Q-Pulse. It is then reviewed and approved by the section lead and quality manager before being released to all staff. The old version is automatically archived, preventing any outdated instructions from being used.

Question 194:

Can you tell us about error logging and incident reporting in the laboratory?

Answer:

Error logging usually refers to recording minor or routine mistakes that occur in the laboratory. for example, a QC failure, sample mislabelling caught before reporting, or an analyser error that was corrected before results were released. These are documented to monitor trends and prevent recurrence. Incident reporting, on the other hand, refers to more significant events such as reporting an incorrect result, equipment failure affecting patient results, or a breach of sample traceability. These incidents require a formal investigation, often including root cause analysis, corrective and preventive actions (CAPA), and follow-up review by the Quality or Management team.

Error logging and incident reporting are essential parts of the laboratory's quality management system. They allow us to identify, record, and investigate any errors, near-misses, or non-conformances that could affect the accuracy of results or patient safety.

In our laboratory, all incidents are recorded through the Q-Pulse quality management system. Each report includes details such as what happened, when and where it occurred, who was involved, and any immediate corrective actions taken. The Quality Team or section lead then carries out a root cause analysis to understand why it happened and implements corrective and preventive actions to stop it from recurring.

We also categorise incidents by their severity, for example sample labelling errors, equipment failures, or incorrect result entry, and review trends during audit meetings or management reviews. This helps us to learn from mistakes and continuously improve our processes.

Ultimately, error logging and incident reporting are not about blaming individuals, but about maintaining transparency, learning from issues, and safeguarding patient care.

For example, we once logged a sample mislabelling incident **in Blood Transfusion**. After investigation, we found that the issue arose from confusion during ward labelling. As a corrective action, we arranged refresher training for ward staff and updated our sample acceptance SOP. This improved compliance and reduced similar incidents.

Question 195:

Can you explain internal and external audits in the laboratory?

Answer:

Audits are systematic checks to ensure that laboratory processes, procedures, and systems are compliant with standards, accurate, and safe. They help identify areas for improvement, prevent errors, and ensure the lab is operating according to its Quality Management System."

Internal Audits:

Internal audits are carried out by the laboratory itself, usually by trained staff who are independent of the area being audited. The aim is to monitor compliance with SOPs, policies, ISO 15189 standards, and internal procedures.

Internal audits might cover areas like document control, equipment maintenance, IQC performance, or staff competencies. Findings are documented, corrective actions assigned, and follow-up checks are performed to ensure improvements are implemented. Internal audits help the lab proactively identify and fix issues before they affect patient care or an external assessment.

External Audits:

External audits are carried out by outside bodies, such as UKAS assessors, regulatory authorities, or peer reviewers. The aim is to independently verify that the laboratory meets accreditation standards and regulatory requirements.

External audits assess both management and technical aspects, including sample handling, testing processes, QC records, staff competence, and overall compliance with ISO 15189. Any non-conformities identified must be addressed, with evidence of corrective actions provided. External audits provide assurance to patients, clinicians, and regulators that the laboratory delivers safe, reliable, and high-quality results.

In our Biochemistry department, internal audits are scheduled quarterly. For example, we audit analyser QC documentation and staff competency records. Findings are logged in Q-Pulse and corrective actions are tracked. During a recent UKAS external audit, these records were reviewed and confirmed to meet ISO 15189 standards, which helped maintain our accreditation.

Question 196:

What is the difference between a QC shift and a trend?

Answer:

Shifts show sudden, consecutive deviation and Trends show gradual deviation over time. However, both shifts and trends are patterns seen in internal quality control (IQC) data and identifying them is essential for detecting errors in laboratory testing.

QC Shift:

Definition: A shift occurs when several consecutive QC results fall consistently above or below the mean (typically 6 or more consecutive points).

Indicates: A sudden change in the analytical system. For example, a reagent change, calibration error, analyser malfunction, or lot variation.

Action: Investigate immediately, check the analyser, recalibrate if needed, and repeat QC before releasing patient results.

QC Trend:

Definition: A trend occurs when QC results gradually move in one direction over time, either increasing or decreasing relative to the mean.

Indicates: A slow deterioration of the system. For example, reagent degradation, instrument drift, or gradual wear of analyser components.

Action: Investigate the cause, perform maintenance or recalibration, and monitor closely until the trend stabilises.

For example, **in Biochemistry**, if six consecutive glucose QC results are above the mean after a new reagent lot is introduced, that's a shift and we would immediately investigate before reporting patient results. If the QC values slowly increase over two weeks, that's a trend indicating possible analyser drift, requiring maintenance and close monitoring.

Question 197:

Describe the qualities that a senior biomedical scientist should have.

Answer:

A senior biomedical scientist should combine technical expertise with leadership, communication, and managerial skills to ensure the laboratory runs efficiently and safely.

Key Qualities:

1. **Technical Competence and Knowledge:**

- Expert understanding of laboratory techniques, instrumentation, and quality standards.
- Able to troubleshoot complex issues and mentor junior staff.

2. **Leadership and Team Management:**

- Guides and supports the team, delegates tasks appropriately, and motivates staff.
- Promotes a positive and collaborative working environment.

3. **Communication Skills:**

- Clear and effective communication with colleagues, clinicians, and multidisciplinary teams.
- Able to explain complex results or problems in understandable terms.

4. **Decision-Making and Problem-Solving:**

- Able to make timely, informed decisions, especially during incidents, equipment downtime, or unexpected results.
- Uses evidence and protocols to guide actions.

5. **Quality and Safety Focus:**

- Ensures compliance with SOPs, ISO 15189, and UKAS standards.
- Monitors IQC/EQA, audits, and incident reports to maintain high-quality service.

6. **Organisational and Planning Skills:**

- Prioritises workload, manages resources effectively, and ensures smooth workflow.
- Balances managerial responsibilities with technical duties.

7. **Mentorship and Staff Development:**

- Trains, supervises, and develops junior staff, ensuring competence and confidence.
- Supports CPD and career development.

8. **Adaptability and Resilience:**

- Able to manage unexpected challenges, such as staff shortages, high workload, or system failures.
- Maintains professionalism under pressure.

Example: In my current role, I supervise junior staff while managing IQC and EQA reporting. I also handle equipment downtime by delegating tasks, coordinating with colleagues, and ensuring that patient results are still delivered safely and on time. This requires a combination of technical knowledge, leadership, and organisation.

Question 198:

What is accuracy and precision and how can you differentiate the two?

Answer:

What is accuracy and precision, and how can you differentiate between the two?"

Accuracy and precision are both measures of laboratory test performance, but they describe different aspects of reliability.

Accuracy

Definition: Accuracy refers to how close a measured result is to the true or reference value.

Focus: Correctness of the result.

Example: If a patient's glucose level is actually 5.5 mmol/L, and your analyser reads 5.4 mmol/L, the measurement is accurate. Because 5.4 mmol/L result is close to 5.5 mmol/L, which is the actual value. That makes it accurate.

Precision

Definition: Precision refers to the repeatability or reproducibility of measurements, which is how close repeated measurements are to each other, regardless of whether they are close to the true value.

Focus: Consistency of results.

Example: If repeated glucose measurements of the same sample are 5.0, 5.1, 5.0, and 5.1 mmol/L, the test is precise, even if the true value is 5.5 mmol/L. Meaning that if it was 5.0, 4.0, 3.0, 6.0 mmol/L, the test result is not precise.

In Biochemistry, Haematology, and other disciplines, we monitor both accuracy and precision using Internal Quality Control (IQC) and External Quality Assessment (EQA). IQC helps detect issues with precision, such as random variation, while EQA compares our results against a reference or peer group to assess accuracy. Both are essential to ensure patient results are reliable and safe for clinical decision-making.

Question 199:

What is systematic and random error, and how can you differentiate the two?

Answer:

In laboratory testing, errors can broadly be classified into systematic and random errors. Both affect the reliability of results, but in different ways.

Systematic Error (Bias)

Definition: A consistent, reproducible error that shifts all results in the same direction from the true value.

Effect: Affects accuracy, not precision.

Cause: Faulty calibration, incorrect reagent, incorrect technique, or instrument malfunction.

Example: If a glucose analyser consistently reads 0.5 mmol/L higher than the true value, that's a systematic error.

Detection: EQA (External Quality Assessment) or comparison with reference methods like laboratories cross check.

Random Error

Definition: Unpredictable variations that occur occasionally in measurements.

Effect: Affects precision, not accuracy.

Cause: Small fluctuations in instrument performance, environmental conditions, or operator technique.

Example: Repeated measurements of the same glucose sample might give 5.0, 5.1, 5.0, 5.2 mmol/L.

Detection: Internal QC (repeating measurements and checking for consistency).

In Biochemistry, systematic errors are identified through EQA or cross-checking with a reference method, while random errors are monitored by IQC to ensure repeatability. Both need to be managed carefully to ensure patient results are safe, reliable, and trustworthy.

Question 200:

Would you say you have had a good interview today?

Answer 1:

Yes, thank you. I feel it has been a productive discussion, and I have enjoyed the opportunity to talk about my experience and how I can contribute to the team. It has also given me a clearer picture of the Trust and the department, which makes me even more enthusiastic about this role.

Answer 2:

I think it has gone well. I have been able to discuss my experience and the ways I can support quality and patient care in the laboratory. Of course, I always reflect afterwards to see if there are areas I could explain more clearly, but overall, I have found it very positive.

Question 201:

If you are not successful for this position, would you be happy for us to keep your details on file for future opportunities within the Trust?

Answer 1:

Yes, absolutely. I would very much appreciate that. I am genuinely interested in working within this Trust because I share its values and I am enthusiastic about the quality of work and learning opportunities here. Even if I am not successful this time, I would be keen to be considered for future roles where my skills and experience could contribute to the team.

Answer 2:

Thank you for the opportunity to interview today. I have really enjoyed discussing how my skills and experience can contribute to the team and the Trust's values of quality, safety, and patient care. I am genuinely interested in being part of your laboratory, and even if I am not successful this time, I would be very happy for my details to be kept on record for future opportunities. I appreciate your time and consideration.

Question 202:

Can you tell me the recent ISO 15189:2022 changes?

Answer:

The international standard ISO 15189 specifies the requirements for quality and competence in medical laboratories. The most recent update, ISO 15189:2022, replaced ISO 15189:2012 and was published in December 2022. Laboratories accredited to the 2012 version are required to transition to the 2022 version within the defined timeframe set by their national accreditation body (for example, UKAS in the United Kingdom).This question tests your understanding of key changes introduced in ISO 15189:2022, their impact on laboratory operations, and your ability to relate them to real-world pathology practice.

You are expected to show that you:

- Understand the major revisions made in ISO 15189:2022 compared to ISO 15189:2012.
- Can explain how the changes affect laboratory quality systems, patient safety, and daily operations.
- Are able to apply the changes practically across pathology disciplines such as haematology, microbiology, biochemistry, and histopathology.
- Know about the importance of transition planning and staff training.

Answer:

The release of ISO 15189:2022 introduced several significant changes designed to strengthen patient safety, risk management, and integration of modern laboratory practices.

Stronger focus on patient-centred risk management:

The new version emphasises risk-based thinking across all stages of testing such as pre-analytical, analytical, and post-analytical. Laboratories must identify, assess, and mitigate risks that could impact patient safety or test validity. For example, **in haematology,** if an analyser drifts in calibration, the laboratory must document the issue, assess how it could have affected patient results (e.g., delayed or incorrect transfusion decisions), and take preventive actions.

Inclusion of Point-of-Care Testing (POCT) requirements:

The new standard now incorporates requirements for POCT, previously covered separately under ISO 22870. This means POCT must follow the same quality and competence framework as core laboratory testing. For example, **in microbiology**, if rapid antigen or molecular POCT devices are used for infectious disease screening, they must undergo validation, operator training, and ongoing QC/EQA monitoring under the same governance as central lab instruments.

Structural and terminology updates:

ISO 15189:2022 has been reorganised to align with other ISO standards such as ISO/IEC 17025. Management and technical requirements have been streamlined for clarity. For example, **in biochemistry,** documentation such as method validation, equipment calibration, and measurement uncertainty must now be clearly traceable under technical sections rather than dispersed throughout quality documents.

Enhanced competence, authorisation, and method verification:

The standard reinforces the need for formal staff competence assessment, authorisation for tasks, and robust verification or validation of all methods used. For example**, in histopathology**, introducing a new digital pathology workflow would require validation of image quality, verification of diagnostic accuracy, and formal authorisation for staff before implementation.

Transition and accreditation timelines:

Accreditation bodies require all laboratories to complete the transition from ISO 15189:2012 to ISO 15189:2022 by a specified date. For example, UKAS states that as of 1 January 2024 assessments will be to ISO 15189:2022 and by 6 December 2025 accreditation to the 2012 version will cease. Also, Quality Managers must perform a gap analysis, update quality documentation, train staff, and demonstrate compliance at their next assessment visit. For example, a lab's Quality Manager must undertake a gap analysis versus ISO 15189:2022, prepare a transition plan, update its QMS, SOPs, Policies, risk register, train staff, and submit evidence ahead of their next surveillance assessment.

Conclusion:

ISO 15189:2022 represents a modernised, risk-based, patient-centred approach to medical laboratory quality. It integrates POCT oversight, strengthens competence and method verification, and aligns better with international quality management principles. As a biomedical scientist, my understanding and applying these changes means ensuring that every aspect of laboratory practice from sample receipt to result reporting promotes patient safety, traceability, and continuous improvement. This knowledge demonstrates my knowledge of these updates and highlight both my professional awareness and readiness to work in an accredited, quality-driven environment.

Appendix

Supporting Information Template (Please don't plagiarise – Just use as a guide)

Dear Hiring Manager,

I am writing to express my keen interest in the Pathology Quality Manager/Training Co-ordinator. With over twelve years of experience in pathology laboratories, I have honed my skills in various areas such as Haematology, and Blood Transfusion. My journey in the field began with my undergraduate studies in Medical Laboratory Science at Imo State University, Nigeria, where my passion for biomedical science flourished through years of dedication and enthusiasm.

I am a dedicated Biomedical Scientist (BMS) with a keen eye for detail and a strong commitment to excellence. Over the course of my career, I have had the opportunity to work across various pathology units, gaining valuable experience in both manual analysis and automation. My ability to quickly grasp new skills and knowledge has allowed me to adapt seamlessly to evolving demands and take on challenging roles with confidence. In my role, I have operated a wide range of equipment, including Cobas 501, 601, and 6000 for biochemistry, Sysmex XN line and Beckman Coulter DxH for full blood count and thin film, Sysmex C5-2100i and TOP550 for coagulation profiles, OrthoVision and IH-1000 for blood group and antibody screening, Vitek for sensitivity testing, and Bactech alert for blood culture. Additionally, I am proficient in utilizing Cobas x480 for Chlamydia analysis. My experience spans across disciplines such as Haematology, Blood Transfusion, Microbiology, and Biochemistry. However, my current area of specialty is haematology and blood transfusion.

My continuous pursuit of skill acquisition and knowledge enhancement has enabled me to excel in the computerized laboratory environment, where I am comfortable working independently and without supervision. I have also undergone training in the national laboratory accreditation process, gaining valuable insights into quality management systems, including proper documentation, reagent and analyzer validation, error logging, DATIX incidence reporting and investigation, IQM SOP Draft, IQM SOP Revision, and corrective and preventive actions (CAPA). My strong verbal and written communication skills, coupled with proficiency in computer systems and applications, have allowed me to effectively collaborate with colleagues and serve as a source of inspiration within the team.

My tenure in pathology laboratories has provided me with extensive experience and insight into the dynamic nature of the Biomedical Science profession. Throughout my career, I have witnessed numerous changes and advancements driven by ongoing research and innovation. These developments have required continuous adaptation and learning, as new guidelines and technologies continue to reshape laboratory practice.

The advent of automation has been a significant catalyst for change, revolutionising biomedical science and enhancing diagnostic capability. Automation has not only expedited diagnostic processes, reducing turnaround times and supporting timely patient care, but has also expanded the responsibilities of Biomedical Scientists. With the integration of automated analysers, our role has evolved to include greater organisational and managerial responsibility, including overseeing workflows and training staff in the use of advanced technologies.

While automation has streamlined many aspects of laboratory work, it has also introduced new challenges, particularly in ensuring the reliability and reproducibility of results. As a Biomedical Scientist, I remain vigilant in verifying and validating automated processes, recognising the importance of mitigating potential risks to patient safety and maintaining the highest standards of quality.

Furthermore, effective communication skills have emerged as indispensable assets in our role as Biomedical Scientists. Clear and concise communication is essential for training colleagues in the use of new technologies, as well as for disseminating vital information to the public. By fostering open dialogue and knowledge sharing, I have a good communication skill, which contributes to my ability to uphold the quality of services provided in the pathology laboratory and contribute to the advancement of the profession.

I am a HCPC registered Biomedical Scientist and a Fellow member of Institute of Biomedical Science (FIBMS) with more than twelve (12) years' experience in pathology laboratory. I am competent in sample analysis, analysers troubleshooting, use and application of laboratory information system (LIMs) to validate results. I have good analytical skills and practical pathology laboratory experience. Following the completion of my undergraduate studies, I was awarded a Bachelor of Science degree in Medical Laboratory Science, which is equivalent to a Biomedical Science degree accredited by the Institute of Biomedical Science (IBMS) in the UK. Since then, I have worked in a reputable hospital, which enhanced my pathology laboratory experiences. While working in these hospitals, I have had the opportunity to expand my experience in Haematology and Blood Bank.

My understanding of International Organizational Standardization (ISO) and the United Kingdom Accreditation Service (UKAS), coupled with my commitment to quality within a pathology laboratory, has been the driving force behind my efforts to improve laboratory processes to meet ISO standards. I have demonstrated this commitment in my workplace through my organizational and management abilities, as well as my experience in inventory management of laboratory commodities, laboratory safety, and quality management systems (QMS). I actively participated in quality control (QC) testing and External Quality Assessment (EQA) procedures, ensuring the accuracy and reliability of laboratory results.

Furthermore, I possess expertise in manual testing procedures such as ABO/Rh Card grouping, IgG card antibody screening, and Card Phenotyping, among others. I am skilled in conducting various tests including the Direct antiglobulin test (DAT), Indirect antiglobulin test (IAT), manual Erythrocyte Sedimentation Rate (ESR), and Prothrombin Time (PT) analysis, among others. Additionally, I am proficient in techniques such as blood

Crossmatching, biological sample culture, and isolation and identification of microorganisms. My proficiency with microscope applications further enhances my capabilities for a range of identification and analysis tasks. I possess a thorough understanding of consumables and reagents management, including the crucial tasks of reagent verification and validation. Additionally, I am well-versed in the development and documentation of standard operating procedures (SOPs) and adept at reporting incidents as per established protocols.

Continuing to advance my career as a biomedical scientist has always been a priority for me, which is why I am applying for the Section Manager/Trainee - Haematology position at your reputable hospital. I believe that working in your institution will provide me with the opportunity to contribute to the team and the overall goals of the department while furthering my professional development.

Having carefully reviewed the job description and person specification for this role, I am confident that my skills, qualities, qualifications, and experiences align closely with the requirements outlined. Additionally, I resonate with the values upheld by the organization, which further strengthens my desire to work in this environment.

Thank you for considering my application. I am eager to have the opportunity to contribute to your team and engage in further discussions regarding how I can support the goals of the department.

Sincerely,

Dr Emmanuel Ogbodo

www.ingramcontent.com/pod-product-compliance
Lightning Source LLC
LaVergne TN
LVHW070827220926
848486LV00028B/94